WHAT THEY DIDN'T TELL YOU IN SCHOOL

A Real-World Guide to Entrepreneurship, Corporate America, and Owning Your Future

Thomas Hightower

This book is dedicated to my daughters, **Gianna and Ava Hightower**. May you always believe in yourselves more than the world doubts you, and may you never be afraid to chase the life God placed on your hearts.

To my entire family for your love, sacrifices, and unwavering support. This journey would not be possible without you.

To the great mentors and teachers who guided me, challenged me, and pushed me to become better than I thought I could be—thank you for seeing potential before results.

And above all, to my Lord and Savior **Jesus Christ**, for the strength when I was weak, the faith when the path was unclear, and the purpose behind every step of this journey. All glory belongs to You.

TABLE OF CONTENTS

FOREWORD

Read This Before You Do Anything Else

Let me talk to you for a moment—not like a teacher, not like a coach, not like someone trying to impress you but like someone who has been where you are. Because before you read another word, you need to understand this: **You did not pick up this book by accident**. People don't just "stumble" into moments like this. You're here because something inside you knows there's more—more than your current situation, more than what people expect of you, and more than what life has shown you so far.

Maybe you can't explain it yet. Maybe you don't have the words. Maybe all you have is a feeling—a tension in your chest, a frustration that won't go away, a hunger that doesn't shut off. That feeling is not random. That feeling is potential knocking. Potential is dangerous if you ignore it. I know because I almost did.

The Voices That Try to Decide Your Future

When I was at Stafford High, people were very comfortable telling me what I *couldn't* do.

Not quietly.

Not carefully.

Out loud.

Repeatedly.

"You're not D1 material."

"You're barely passing."

"You're not university-bound."

"Be realistic."

"You come from a small school in a small town."

They said it like they were helping me. Like they were protecting me from disappointment. But what they were really doing was handing me a smaller version of life and hoping I'd accept it. And here's the truth no one says out loud:

Most people don't doubt you because you're incapable.

They doubt you because your ambition threatens their comfort.

They had already decided what was "possible"—and anything outside of that made them uneasy. So, they tried to make *me* smaller. But something inside me wouldn't let that sit right.

The Room Where Everything Changed

Every night, I'd go home to my room. That room wasn't special. That house wasn't fancy. But those walls? Those walls told a different story. They were covered with posters of universitiesschools people told me were unrealistic. Places people said I didn't belong. Futures people thought were out of reach. And I'd stand there, alone, staring at them. I was not wishing, not hoping, I was **Believing**—believing in a version of myself no one else could see yet. That's when I learned one of the most important lessons of my life:

People judge you by where you are.

You must commit to where you're going.

They saw my grades.

They saw my environment.

They saw my limitations.

I saw possibility. And belief—real belief—changes how you move through the world.

What School Never Prepared You For

School teaches you how to pass tests. It does NOT teach you
- how to handle doubt
- how to recover from failure
- how to manage pressure
- how to build confidence
- how to create opportunity
- how to believe in yourself when no one else does.

School rewards compliance.

Life rewards ownership.

And the moment you step out into the real world, you realize something terrifying:

Nobody is coming to save you.

Not your teachers.

Not your parents.

Not your friends.

Not your boss.

The world does not care how much potential you have if you never use it. That realization either breaks people…or it wakes them up. This book exists to wake you up.

Why This Book Is Different

This is not a theory. This is not "feel good" motivation that fades by Monday morning. This book is built from doubt, failure, discipline, real decisions, uncomfortable growth, and ownership. It's built for people who feel behind, for people who feel underestimated, and for people who know they have more in them but don't yet know how to unlock it.

And listen carefully:

You do not need to have it all figured out to start.
You just need to be honest enough to grow.
That's it.

A Warning Before You Continue

If you want comfort, stop here. If you want excuses, this book isn't for you. If you want someone to blame for where you are, this book will frustrate you. Because this book will challenge you to take responsibility—not someday, not later, but now. It will ask you to do the following:

- Look at your habits.
- Question your mindset.
- Evaluate your environment.
- Confront your discipline.
- Raise your standards.

That's uncomfortable.
But discomfort is the price of becoming someone you respect.

The Promise

If you read this book fully—not passively, not casually, but intentionally—you will not be the same person at the end.
You will

- think differently
- move differently
- expect more from yourself
- tolerate less nonsense
- take ownership of your future.

Not because life suddenly gets easier—but because **you get stronger**.

And once that happens?

Nothing can take that from you.

One Last Thing

Before you turn the page, I want you to say this—out loud if you can:

"I'm done playing small. I'm ready to build."

Good. Let's get to work.

INTRODUCTION

WHAT THEY DIDN'T TELL YOU IN SCHOOL

Let's start with the truth. School did not fail you—but it did not prepare you either. That's hard for some people to hear, especially if you were told from a young age that education was the key to everything. "Do well in school and you'll be set." "Get good grades and life will work out." "Go to college and success will follow." That message sounds good. It just isn't complete. Because the moment you step out of school—high school, college, or even grad school—reality hits you fast. And when it does, you realize something uncomfortable: **The rules changed…and no one told you.** The real world doesn't hand out syllabi.

It doesn't give you extra credit.

It doesn't curve the test.

It doesn't care how hard you *tried*.

It cares about what you can do, how you think, how you respond to pressure, and whether you can take responsibility when things don't go your way. And that's where a lot of young people get stuck.

The Shock After School

I've seen it over and over. Smart students who feel lost. Good kids who feel behind. Talented people who feel invisible. They followed the rules. They did what they were told. They checked the boxes. And yet, here they are—unsure, overwhelmed, and questioning themselves. Not because they're lazy. Not because they're dumb. Not because they lack potential. But because **no one ever taught them how life actually works**. School taught you

- how to memorize
- how to repeat information
- how to raise your hand
- how to follow instructions.

It did not teach you

- how to believe in yourself
- how to manage fear
- how to handle rejection
- how to communicate under pressure
- how to make decisions without approval
- how to fail and get back up
- how to build confidence when results aren't there yet.

Those skills are not optional.
They are survival skills.

The Gap No One Talks About

There is a massive gap between education and execution, knowing and doing, potential and performance, and between ambition and reality. School lives on one side of that gap. Life lives on the other. And if no one shows you how to cross it, you end up standing in the middle—confused, frustrated, and doubting yourself. I know that feeling personally. Growing up in Stafford, I was constantly told to lower my expectations. Not in a cruel way—in a "realistic" way. But realism, when it's rooted in fear, is just another form of limitation. People weren't asking me what I wanted. They were telling me what they thought was possible. And that's dangerous. Because when you're young, you don't just hear those messages—you absorb them. You start questioning yourself. You start shrinking your goals. You start settling before life even asks you to. This book exists to interrupt that process.

Why Talent Isn't Enough

One of the biggest lies school accidentally teaches is this: "If you're smart or talented, you'll be fine." That's not how the world works. Talent without discipline dies. Intelligence without confidence stalls. Potential without execution expires. I've seen incredibly gifted people waste years of their life waiting to feel "ready." I've also seen average people build extraordinary lives because they learned how to

- show up consistently
- learn fast
- adapt
- Recieve feedback
- own their mistakes
- stay disciplined when motivation fades.

The world rewards **ownership**, not excuses. And school doesn't train you for ownership—it trains you for instruction. That's why the transition feels so jarring.

Corporate America, Entrepreneurship, and Real Life

Here's another truth they didn't tell you: Corporate America is a game.

Entrepreneurship is a responsibility. Life is a pressure test. None of them care how uncomfortable you feel. In corporate environments, nobody walks you step by step once you're in. You're expected to figure things out, advocate for yourself, communicate clearly, and produce results. In entrepreneurship, nobody saves you. No paycheck shows up unless you earn it. No structure exists unless you build it. No one tells you what to do—which sounds exciting until it's terrifying. And in life? Life doesn't pause because you're unsure.

Bills still come. Expectations still rise. Time keeps moving. That's why mindset matters more than credentials.

What This Book Will Actually Teach You

This book is not here to motivate you for a day. It's here to **retrain how you think**.

You'll learn

- how to turn doubt into fuel instead of fear
- how to build belief before results show up
- how to develop discipline when motivation disappears
- how to navigate corporate spaces strategically
- how to approach entrepreneurship realistically
- how to protect your energy and environment
- how to own your future instead of waiting for permission.

This book will challenge you to stop asking, *"What should I do?"* and start asking, *"Who do I need to become?"* Because your outcomes will always reflect your identity.

This Book Is a Conversation, Not a Lecture

I'm not writing this from a pedestal. I'm writing this from experience.

From being doubted.

From being underestimated.

From not having a clear roadmap.

From having to figure things out the hard way.

You don't need perfection.

You don't need all the answers.

You don't need confidence yet.

You need honesty.

Honesty about where you are.

Honesty about your habits.

Honesty about your excuses.

Honesty about your potential.

That's where growth starts.

One Decision That Changes Everything

At some point—and this is the moment that separates people—you must decide the following: Am I going to keep waiting…or am I going to take ownership? Because nobody hands you belief. Nobody hands you discipline. Nobody hands you confidence. You build those. And once you do, everything changes.

Read This Book the Right Way

Don't rush this. Don't skim.

Pause.

Reflect.

Write things down.

Apply what hits you.
Growth doesn't come from reading—it comes from action.

Final Word Before Chapter 1

You are not behind. You are not broken. You are not late. You are early—if you decide to take control now. This book is not here to save you. It's here to **hand you the tools**. What you build with them is up to you.

CHAPTER 1

TURNING DOUBT INTO FUEL

How to Use What Was Meant to Break You to Build You

Doubt doesn't ask permission. It shows up early. It shows up loud. And it almost always shows up right when you start believing in yourself. That's not an accident. Doubt follows potential. If no one ever doubted you, it wouldn't mean you're special—it would mean you're staying safely inside expectations. Doubt shows up when you step outside of what people are comfortable with. I learned that lesson early.

When Doubt Comes from People You Expect to Believe in You

At Stafford High, doubt wasn't subtle. It didn't come from strangers online or people who didn't know me. It came from places that were supposed to build me.

Teachers.

Coaches.

Adults who meant well.

Peers who thought they were being "real."

"You're not D1 material."

"You're not university-bound."

"You're barely passing."

"You should have a backup plan."

At first, I didn't know what to do with those words. Because when authority figures speak, you assume they're right. You assume they see something you don't. You assume they're telling you the truth. That's the dangerous part of doubt—when it comes wrapped as advice. Most people don't doubt you maliciously. They doubt you **confidently**. And confidence makes doubt sound believable. If you're young, this is where dreams quietly die—not because people scream at you but because they calmly convince you to lower your expectations.

The Moment Doubt Becomes Internal

The real problem isn't what people say. The real problem is what happens **after** they say it. Because doubt doesn't destroy you on impact—it destroys you when you replay it.

You hear it once…

then again in your head…

then again when you fail…

then again when you're tired…

then again when results don't show up fast enough.

Before you realize it, doubt isn't outside anymore. It's inside. And once doubt lives inside you, it starts shaping your decisions. You stop raising your hand. You stop applying. You stop trying as hard. You stop believing effort will matter. Not because you gave up but because you adjusted your expectations to avoid disappointment. That's how potential gets buried quietly.

The Night I Decided Doubt Wouldn't Decide for Me

There was a night I still remember clearly. I came home after another long day of being reminded of everything I "wasn't." I walked into my room, shut the door, and stood there staring at the posters on my wall—universities people said were unrealistic, dreams people thought were embarrassing, goals people didn't take seriously. And standing there, something clicked. Not motivation. Not confidence. Clarity. I realized something simple but powerful: **If I let other people decide what was possible for me, I would never forgive myself.** I didn't suddenly become great that night. But I made a decision: Doubt was no longer a verdict. It was information. And information can be used.

The Difference Between Doubt and Truth

Here's something no one explains when you're young: Doubt is loud. Truth is quiet. Doubt speaks in absolutes: "You'll never." "You can't." "You're not built for this." Truth speaks in possibilities: "You can grow." "You can learn." "You're not done yet." Doubt focuses on where you are. Truth focuses on what's possible with effort. Once I understood that, doubt stopped scaring me. Doubt wasn't predicting my future—it was reacting to my potential.

How to Turn Doubt Into Fuel (The Real Way)

Most people hear "use doubt as fuel" and think it means getting angry or proving people wrong publicly. That's not how it works. Real fuel doesn't burn outward—it burns inward. Here's how you use doubt.

1. Stop arguing with it.

You don't win by convincing people. You win by becoming undeniable. Every minute you spend explaining yourself is energy taken away from building yourself. Silence + work = power.

2. Translate doubt into direction.

When someone doubts you, ask the following: What do I need to improve? What skill am I missing? What habit is weak? Where am I undisciplined? Doubt reveals gaps. Gaps give you a plan.

3. Use repetition to build confidence.

Confidence doesn't come from believing harder. It comes from doing the work repeatedly. When you train consistently—when you study when it's boring or show up, when you're tired—confidence grows naturally. And once confidence grows, doubt loses leverage.

The Moment You Stop Needing Permission

Here's the shift that changes everything: At some point, you stop asking, "Do you think I can?" And you start asking, "What do I need to do?" That's when doubt stops controlling you. Doubt feeds on hesitation. Decisive people are hard to shake.

Why Doubt Will Follow You Your Entire Life

Let me be clear doubt doesn't disappear when you succeed. It just changes form. People will doubt

- your leadership
- your growth
- your ideas
- your consistency
- your next level.

That's not a sign you're failing. It's a sign you're still growing. The goal isn't to eliminate doubt. The goal is to **outgrow it**.

The Real Win

The real win isn't proving people wrong. The real win is becoming someone who no longer needs validation, someone who knows who they are, where they're going, and what they're willing to do to get there.

When you reach that point, doubt becomes background noise. It doesn't disappear—it just loses power.

Action Steps—Chapter 1

Do not skip this.

1. Write down the top three doubts placed on you.
Be honest. Write them exactly as you've heard them.

2. Identify what each doubt is really pointing to.
A skill gap? A habit issue? A discipline problem?

3. Create a simple plan.
One action per doubt. No overthinking.

4. Do something daily that contradicts the doubt.
Small actions. Consistent effort.

5. Say this daily—out loud.
"Doubt does not decide my future. My actions do."

Final Word for This Chapter

Doubt didn't come to destroy you. It came to test whether you're serious. And now that you know that? Use it.

CHAPTER 2

THE POWER OF BELIEF

Why You Must Believe in Yourself
Long Before the World Does

Belief is where everything starts. Not success. Not confidence. Not opportunity. **Belief.**

Before you ever win externally, you must win internally. And most people never do—not because they can't but because no one ever taught them how. They wait. They wait for confidence to show up. They wait for proof. They wait for permission. They wait for validation. And while they wait, life keeps moving. Belief doesn't wait. Belief decides.

Why Belief Is Harder than People Admit

People love talking about belief when things are going well. It's easy to believe when

- results are showing
- People are cheering
- Progress is visible
- confidence feels natural.

But belief matters **before** all of that. Belief matters when
- you're failing
- you're behind
- you're embarrassed
- you're unsure
- you're doubting yourself.

That's when belief becomes real.

When I was at Stafford High, there was no evidence I was "supposed" to make it. No obvious proof. No guarantees. No roadmap. What I had instead was an inner voice—quiet, stubborn, relentless—that kept saying, **"Don't quit. You're not done."** That voice didn't make sense on paper. But belief rarely does.

The World Will Not Believe in You First

This is a hard truth, but it will save you years of frustration: **The world does not believe in potential. The world believes in results.** That means if you're waiting for belief from teachers, bosses, friends, or family before you commit to yourself—you will wait forever. People believe *after* you succeed. They applaud *after* you win. They support *after* you prove it. Belief always comes last from the outside. It must come first from the inside. I had to learn that early. Because every time I looked for reassurance, I came up empty. Every time I waited for encouragement, it was inconsistent. Every time I asked for validation, it was conditional. So, I stopped asking. And that's when belief began to grow.

Belief Is Not Confidence

This is where most people get confused. Belief is not confidence. Confidence is how you feel. Belief is what you decide. You can believe while feeling insecure. You can believe while being afraid. You can believe while doubting yourself. Belief says, "I'll keep going even if I don't feel ready." Confidence says, "I feel ready now." If you wait for confidence, you'll never start. Belief allows you to move *before* confidence shows up. And movement creates confidence.

The Three Enemies of Belief

If belief is so powerful, why do so many people struggle with it? Because belief is constantly under attack. Here are the three biggest enemies of belief:

1. Your Past

Your past will try to convince you that it defines you. Past mistakes. Past failures. Past grades. Past decisions. Belief requires you to accept this truth:

Your past explains you—it does not limit you.

Growth begins when you stop asking, "What did I do wrong?" and start asking, "What can I do differently?"

2. Your Environment

If you're surrounded by people who settle, complain, quit, and mock ambition, belief becomes harder. Not impossible—but harder. Your environment shapes what feels "normal." And belief often requires you to live *above* what's normal around you. That's lonely. But it's necessary.

3. Lack of Immediate Results

This is the biggest killer of belief. People believe for a week. Then a month. Then nothing happens. So, they stop. What they don't realize is this:

Belief is tested before it is rewarded.
Always.

How Belief Is Actually Built

Belief is not built through affirmations alone. It's built through **evidence you create for yourself**. Here's how:

1. Keep promises to yourself.
Every time you say you'll do something—and do it—belief grows. Every time you don't—belief weakens. Start small. Belief doesn't need big wins. It needs consistency.

2. Do difficult things on purpose.
Comfort kills belief. Discipline builds it. When you do hard things, wake up early, train when you're tired, study when you're bored, or speak when you're nervous, you send your brain a message: "I can be trusted." That's belief.

3. Stack small wins.
Belief grows through momentum. Small wins compound. Action builds belief. Belief fuels action. That loop changes everything.

The Day Belief Becomes Identity

There's a moment—and you'll feel it—when belief stops being something you practice and starts being who you are.
You stop
- asking for permission
- waiting for approval
- shrinking your goals.

You start
- trusting your decisions
- moving with intention
- owning your direction.

At that point, people notice. Not because you're loud but because you're grounded. And grounded people are dangerous in the best way.

Why Belief Makes People Uncomfortable

Here's something no one prepares you for: When you believe in yourself unapologetically, people react. Some will support you. Some will question you. Some will doubt you harder. Not because you changed but because belief exposes what others lack. Don't dim it. Belief isn't arrogance. It's responsibility.

Belief Is a Daily Practice

Belief is not permanent. You must renew it. Daily. Through action. Through discipline. Through reflection. Through growth. If you stop practicing belief, doubt will happily take its place.

Action Steps—Chapter 2

Do these seriously.

1. Write a belief statement.
Who are you becoming? Write it clearly.

2. Identify one belief that's holding you back.
Challenge it daily.

3. Take one action today aligned with your future self.
No negotiation.

4. Remove one habit that weakens belief.
Discipline creates belief.

5. Say this daily:
"I believe in myself enough to act."

Final Word for This Chapter

Belief is not loud. Belief is not flashy. Belief is quiet consistency, and quiet consistency builds unstoppable lives.

CHAPTER 3

MASTERING YOUR SKILLS

Why Talent Gets You Noticed, but Skill Gets You Paid

There is a lie we grow up believing, and it's one of the most dangerous ones we're ever taught.

The lie is this: *talent is enough.*

From a young age, we praise talent. We reward it in classrooms, on fields, and in conversations. We label people "gifted," "naturals," or "born to do this." We assume that if someone is talented, success will eventually find them.

But the real world doesn't work that way.

Talent might get you noticed. It might open a door. It might buy you a little attention early on. But talent does not guarantee results. Talent does not protect you when pressure hits. And talent alone will not keep you in the room when expectations rise.

Skill will.

School praises talent.

Life rewards skill.

And if you don't understand that early, you'll spend years wondering why effort isn't turning into opportunity.

The Difference Between Potential and Performance

Talent is potential. Skill is applied potential.

Most people confuse the two.

They say things like, "I'm good at this," or "I've always been a natural," or "I don't really have to try that hard." And for a while, that mindset works. Early success often comes easily to talented people. They get praise without preparation. They win without discipline. They're told they're special before they've earned consistency.

But then something happens.

They reach a level where everyone is talented.

At that point, talent stops separating people. The room is full of capable individuals. Everyone was "gifted" somewhere along the way. And now the difference is no longer who *can* do the work, it's who *will* do the work, over and over again, long after the novelty wears off.

That's when skill takes over.

Skill is built quietly. It's built through repetition when no one is watching. It's built through fundamentals, not highlights. It's built through humility—the willingness to admit you're not as good as you could be yet.

Talent wants praise.

Skill wants progress.

And the world pays for progress.

The Truth About Skill No One Likes to Hear

Here's the part people don't want to hear:

Skill takes time.

Not weeks.

Not months.

Years.

And most people quit right before skill starts compounding.

They dabble. They jump. They switch. They chase excitement. They look for the next thing that feels new instead of staying committed to the thing that matters. They confuse movement with progress.

Skill does not care how motivated you feel.

Skill responds to repetition.

That's why people with less talent but more discipline pass people who "had potential" all the time. Consistency beats brilliance when brilliance is inconsistent.

The world is full of former prodigies who never learned how to work.

When Skill Became My Way Out

Growing up in Stafford, I didn't have the luxury of assuming things would just work out for me. I wasn't the most gifted student in the room. I wasn't the most physically dominant athlete. I wasn't walking into spaces with instant credibility. What I did have was an uncomfortable realization that eventually became freeing:

If I mastered my craft, people wouldn't be able to ignore me.

So, I stopped trying to impress. I stopped chasing shortcuts. I stopped worrying about how long it would take. Instead, I started asking better questions.

What skills matter here?

What do the top performers do differently when no one is watching?

Where am I weak—honestly?

What am I avoiding because it's uncomfortable?

Skill begins with honesty. Brutal honesty.

You don't build skill by pretending you're better than you are. You build it by acknowledging where you fall short and committing to close the gap.

Why Skill Builds Real Confidence

A lot of people say they need more confidence. Most of the time, that's not true. What they really need is more competence. Confidence built on hype collapses. Confidence built on skill holds.

When you know you've put in the reps, something changes. You don't need to fake certainty. You don't need to talk louder. You don't need to prove yourself constantly.

You speak differently.

You move differently.

You show up calmer.

You don't panic under pressure.

Skill removes anxiety because preparation replaces fear.

You stop *hoping* you're ready.

You *know* you're ready.

And that quiet confidence is powerful.

Skill Is the Great Equalizer

This chapter matters most if you feel behind.

If you didn't come from money.

If you didn't go to a big-name school.

If you don't have connections.

If you feel like you're starting from the outside looking in.

Skill doesn't care about your background.

Skill is earned.

In corporate America, skill buys leverage. In entrepreneurship, skill buys survival. In life, skill buys options. And people with options don't panic—they pivot.

The moment you develop real skill, you stop begging for opportunities and start creating them.

The Skill Stack That Actually Wins

If you want to win long-term, you can't rely on a single ability. You need a *stack* of skills that work together.

The first category is **hard skills**—what you can do. These are measurable abilities like sales, writing, speaking, analytics, technology, marketing, or operations. Hard skills get you hired. They get you paid. They get you in the door.

The second category is **soft skills**—how you operate. Communication, listening, emotional control, professionalism, adaptability, leadership. You can be technically brilliant and still get passed over if people don't trust you or enjoy working with you.

The third category is **self-management skills**—who you are. Discipline. Focus. Time management. Consistency. Emotional regulation. If you can't manage yourself, nothing else matters.

Most people focus on one category and ignore the rest. That's why progress stalls.

Why Most People Never Master Anything

It's not because they lack ability. It's because they lack patience. People want fast results, visible progress, and early praise. Skill requires repetition without recognition, progress without applause, and effort without guarantees.

Most people quit during the quiet phase—the phase where growth is happening but not visible yet. That's the phase that separates professionals from amateurs.

Skill is built when no one is clapping.

Practice vs. Training

There's a difference between practice and training. Practice repeats what you're comfortable with. Training attacks what you're weak at. Training is uncomfortable. It exposes flaws. It feels slow. That's why it works. If you only do what feels good, you don't grow. If you only train when motivated, you stay average. Skill is built when discipline shows up first.

How to Build Skill Without Burning Out

You don't need obsession. You need structure.

Choose one primary skill. Commit to daily improvement—even thirty focused minutes matters. Track progress weekly. Seek feedback instead of avoiding it. Adjust. Repeat.

Momentum compounds faster than intensity.

When Skill Becomes Identity

At some point, something shifts.

You stop saying, "I'm trying to get better." You start saying, "This is who I am." You don't need hype. You don't need validation. You trust your preparation. Prepared people don't panic.

They perform.

Action Steps

Take this seriously.

Choose one primary skill. One—not five.

Be brutally honest about your current level.

Commit to daily reps, even when it's boring.

Seek feedback instead of avoiding it.
Say this daily: *"I earn my confidence through skill."*

Final Word

Talent is given.
Skill is earned.
And the world will always reward what is earned.

CHAPTER 4

MENTAL TOUGHNESS & RESILIENCE

Why Life Breaks Some People and Builds Others

Life has a way of applying pressure at the exact moment you think you're already carrying enough.

Just when you believe you've figured things out, something shifts. A setback hits. A door closes. A plan falls apart. And suddenly, everything you thought you knew about yourself is tested.

This is where mental toughness shows up—or exposes itself.

Mental toughness isn't something you talk about when things are going well. It's something you discover when they aren't. It reveals itself in moments when quitting feels justified, when slowing down feels reasonable, and when giving up would make perfect sense to everyone watching.

The truth is, life doesn't break people randomly. It applies pressure consistently. And pressure doesn't create character—it reveals it.

The Lie That Life Gets Easier

One of the most dangerous beliefs young people carry is the idea that life eventually "calms down." That once you get past this stage—high school, college, your first job, your first failure—things will finally become manageable.

That belief sets people up for disappointment.

Life doesn't get easier. It gets heavier. Responsibilities increase. Expectations rise. The margin for error shrinks. Pressure doesn't disappear—it changes shape.

What *does* change is your capacity to carry it.

Mental toughness isn't about eliminating stress. It's about increasing your ability to function within it.

What Mental Toughness Actually Is

Mental toughness isn't being emotionless. It's not pretending you don't feel pressure, fear, disappointment, or frustration. Mental toughness is the ability to feel all of that—and still make disciplined decisions. It's staying composed when emotions want to take control. It's choosing long-term growth over short-term relief. It's understanding that how you *respond* matters far more than what happens to you.

Mentally tough people aren't immune to stress. They've simply learned how to manage it instead of being managed by it.

When Quitting Feels Logical

There will be moments in your life when quitting doesn't feel dramatic—it feels practical. Moments when you're tired. When progress feels invisible. When effort doesn't match results. When people start asking, "Why are you still doing this?"

Those are the moments that define resilience.

Resilient people don't always feel strong. They feel committed.

They don't wake up every day inspired. They wake up disciplined.

And more often than not, resilience is built quietly—not in bold declarations but in small decisions like the following:

Just one more day.

Just finish this.

Just don't quit today.

Repeated enough times, those decisions turn into identity.

Resilience Is a Skill, Not a Personality Trait

Some people believe resilience is something you're born with. That certain people are "just built different."

That's not true.

Resilience is trained.

Just like physical strength, mental toughness grows through controlled resistance. Every time you sit in discomfort instead of escaping it, you get stronger. Every time you respond thoughtfully instead of emotionally, your capacity expands.

Avoidance weakens resilience. Exposure builds it.

The Role of Failure in Mental Toughness

Failure is unavoidable. But how you interpret failure determines whether it becomes a lesson or a limitation.

Mentally tough people don't see failure as a verdict. They see it as data.

They ask:

What went wrong?

What can I learn?

What needs to change?

Emotionally fragile people ask:

Why me?

What's wrong with me?

Is this even worth it?

The questions you ask after failure shape the trajectory of your life.

Why Emotional Decisions Are So Costly

Most people don't sabotage themselves through lack of ability. They do it through emotional decision-making.

They quit when they feel discouraged.

They lash out when they feel disrespected.

They procrastinate when they feel overwhelmed.

They settle when they feel tired.

Mental toughness is the ability to pause between feeling and action, to acknowledge emotion without letting it drive the decision. You can feel afraid and still move forward. You can feel uncertain and still commit. You can feel exhausted and still show up.

That's resilience.

Pressure as a Teacher

Pressure isn't personal. It's instructional. It teaches you where your habits are weak. Where your discipline is inconsistent. Where your mindset needs strengthening.

Pressure reveals gaps you wouldn't see otherwise. That's why people who grow learn to stop asking, "Why is this happening to me?" and start asking, "What is this teaching me?"

The lesson may not be comfortable—but it's valuable.

The Three Core Components of Mental Toughness

Mental toughness isn't built randomly. It rests on three foundational elements.

Self-Control

This is the ability to regulate your reactions—to respond instead of reacting, and to keep your composure when emotions spike.

Self-control is power. It allows you to operate strategically instead of impulsively.

Perspective

Without perspective, everything feels overwhelming. Resilient people zoom out. They recognize that most setbacks are temporary, and most problems are survivable.

Perspective doesn't minimize pain—it contextualizes it.

Consistency

Consistency builds stability. When emotions fluctuate, habits carry you forward. Mentally tough people rely on routines when motivation disappears.

Why Comfort Is the Enemy of Resilience

Comfort feels good—but it's deceptive. It convinces you that growth should feel easy. It encourages avoidance. It trains fragility.

Discomfort, on the other hand, forces adaptation. Resilient people intentionally choose discomfort in small doses, so they're prepared when life delivers it unexpectedly.

How Mental Toughness Shows up in Daily Life

Mental toughness isn't dramatic. It's practical.
It looks like the following:
Showing up on time even when no one is watching.
Finishing tasks when motivation fades.
Listening instead of reacting.

Taking responsibility without excuses.

Staying calm under pressure.

These small behaviors compound into strength.

The Confidence That Comes from Resilience

There's a quiet confidence that resilient people carry. Not arrogance. Not bravado. It's the confidence that comes from knowing you've handled difficulty before—and can do it again.

You don't panic as easily.

You don't spiral as quickly.

You trust yourself under pressure.

That trust is earned.

Building Mental Toughness Intentionally

You don't need extreme challenges to build resilience. You need consistency. You need small, intentional practices, such as waking up earlier than comfortably, completing tasks without shortcuts, sitting with difficult conversations, reducing distractions, and following through when it's inconvenient.

Each act strengthens your capacity.

When Life Tests You Again (And It Will)

Resilience isn't a one-time achievement. It's a lifelong practice. Life will test you again.

And again.

And again.

Each test requires a stronger version of you.

The goal isn't to eliminate difficulty. The goal is to become someone who can handle it.

Final Reflection

Mental toughness doesn't make life easier.
It makes *you* stronger.
And strong people don't need life to be easy to move forward.

Action Steps—Chapter 4

1. Identify how you typically respond under pressure.
2. Choose one emotional reaction to improve.
3. Practice controlled discomfort daily.
4. Replace "Why me?" with "What now?"
5. Remind yourself daily: **"Pressure is building me, not breaking me."**

Closing Thought

Resilience is not about surviving life. It's about becoming someone life cannot shake.

CHAPTER 5

SURVIVING AND WINNING IN CORPORATE AMERICA

The Rules Nobody Explains, But Everyone Is Judged By

Corporate America is not what most people think it is. If you were raised to believe that hard work alone guarantees success, this chapter may feel uncomfortable. If you were taught that keeping your head down, doing what you're told, and waiting your turn will eventually pay off, you've likely already felt the confusion and frustration that comes when reality doesn't match the promise.

Corporate America is not school. It does not reward effort the way school does. It rewards results, perception, communication, emotional intelligence, and—whether people want to admit it or not—strategy. Understanding this early can save you years of disappointment.

The First Corporate Shock

Most people enter corporate life optimistic.
They show up early.
They stay late.
They volunteer.

They say yes to everything.

And at first, that effort feels validating. Managers thank them. Teammates appreciate them. Performance reviews are positive.

Then something strange happens. Promotions go to someone else. Opportunities bypass them. Their workload increases—but their influence doesn't. They start asking themselves quiet questions:

Why am I working harder but moving slower?

Why does it feel like others advance without doing more?

What am I missing?

What they're missing is not intelligence or drive. They're missing the rules.

Corporate America Runs on Unwritten Expectations

In school, expectations are clear. You are told what to do, how to do it, and how you'll be graded. In corporate America, expectations are implied. You are evaluated not just on *what* you do, but *how* you do it, *how consistently* you do it, and *how others experience working with you.*

This is where many talented people struggle. They assume performance speaks for itself.

It doesn't.

Performance must be visible, trusted, and aligned with business priorities. You can deliver excellent work and still be overlooked if decision-makers don't understand your impact or don't trust your judgment under pressure.

Your Job Description Is Not Your Value

One of the biggest mindset shifts you must make is separating your title from your contribution. Your job description tells you what you're responsible for. Your value is determined by what problems you solve. The people who rise fastest in corporate environments are not task-completers. They are outcome-owners. They ask better questions.

- What is the real goal here?
- What happens if this fails?
- Who is impacted if this goes wrong?
- How can I make this easier for my manager or my team?

They don't wait to be told what to do next. They anticipate needs. They think beyond their lane. And because of that, leaders begin to trust them with more responsibility.

Why Hard Work Alone Is Not Enough

Hard work is the baseline. Everyone works hard. What separates people is *how* they work. Corporate America rewards people who

- communicate clearly
- manage stress well
- stay composed under pressure
- Take feedback without ego
- understand business priorities.

You can outwork everyone and still lose influence if you lack these skills. This is not unfair—it's functional. Organizations don't promote people who create chaos, confusion, or emotional instability, no matter how talented they are.

The Power of Perception (And Why It Matters)

Perception often gets a bad reputation. People think managing perception means being fake. It doesn't. Managing perception means understanding that people experience you through your actions, communication, and consistency—not your intentions.

Leaders ask themselves the following:

- Can I rely on this person?
- Do they stay calm when things go wrong?
- Do they communicate clearly?
- Do they bring solutions or just problems?

Your answers to those questions shape your trajectory more than your résumé.

Communication Is Your Fastest Leverage

If you want the fastest improvement in your corporate career, improve how you communicate. Clear communication builds trust. Trust creates opportunity. Strong communicators

- summarize instead of ramble
- provide context, not just updates
- anticipate questions
- speak with confidence, not arrogance
- listen as much as they talk.

Poor communication creates doubt—even when the work is good. If leaders don't understand what you're doing, they assume less value than you deserve.

Office Politics: Ignore Them and You Pay the Price

Politics exist in every organization. Not because people are evil—but because humans are involved.

Office politics are really about
- relationships
- influence
- alignment
- trust.

You don't need to gossip. You don't need to manipulate. You *do* need awareness. Know who influences decisions. Understand how priorities are set. Pay attention to how communication flows. Ignoring politics doesn't make you noble—it makes you vulnerable.

Emotional Intelligence Beats Raw Talent

Corporate America is a pressure environment.
Deadlines.
Stakeholders.
Budgets.
Conflicting priorities.
The people who last—and rise—are those who manage themselves well. They don't explode under stress. They don't take feedback personally. They don't make every issue emotional. They stay grounded.
Calm people get trusted. Trusted people get opportunities.

The Danger of "Just Doing Your Job"

Doing what's asked keeps you employed. It does not build influence. People who advance take **intentional ownership**. They
- volunteer strategically
- ask thoughtful questions
- share progress appropriately
- seek feedback proactively.

Not to show off—but to stay aligned with what matters. Visibility without value is noise. Value without visibility is wasted. You need both.

When to Stay and When to Leave

Not every environment is meant to be permanent. Some jobs teach skills. Some teach patience. Some teach boundaries. Staying too long out of fear is just as damaging as leaving too early out of frustration. The key is to make decisions based on growth—not emotion.

Ask yourself:

- Am I learning?
- Am I growing?
- Am I being challenged?
- Am I becoming more capable?

If the answer is no across the board, it may be time to move on.

Corporate America Is a Game—Learn It or Lose to It

This chapter is not here to make you cynical.

It's here to make you prepared.

Corporate America rewards those who understand how it works and move intentionally within it.

You don't need to change who you are.

You need to sharpen how you operate.

Final Word for This Chapter

Corporate America is not unfair. It is **unspoken**. Once you understand the rules, you stop guessing—and start winning.

CHAPTER 6

ENTREPRENEURSHIP: THE REAL WAY

What No One Warns You About
Before You Bet on Yourself

Entrepreneurship has been romanticized to the point of delusion. Scroll through social media long enough, and you'll see the same story repeated over and over: freedom, fast money, flexible schedules, and a life without bosses. The message is seductive—start a business, escape the system, and finally live life on your own terms.

That version of entrepreneurship sells well.

It just isn't real.

The truth is that entrepreneurship is not an escape from responsibility. It is the deepest form of responsibility you will ever take on. There is no syllabus. There is no safety net. There is no one to blame when things don't work.

And that is exactly why most people aren't built for it.

This chapter is not here to hype you up. It's here to tell you the truth—so you don't confuse ambition with readiness, and freedom with avoidance.

Why Most People Want Entrepreneurship for the Wrong Reasons

Many people say they want to be entrepreneurs. What they really want is relief. Relief from bosses. Relief from schedules. Relief from being told what to do. Relief from accountability to someone else.

But entrepreneurship does not remove accountability. It multiplies it. When you work for someone else, your performance affects your paycheck. When you work for yourself, your performance affects everything—your income, your reputation, your stress level, and your future. There is no clocking out mentally. There is no one to hide behind when results aren't there.

Entrepreneurship doesn't ask, *"What do you want?"*

It asks, *"What are you willing to carry?"*

The Loneliness No One Talks About

One of the first surprises for new entrepreneurs is how lonely it feels.

In corporate environments, there is built-in structure. Meetings, colleagues, feedback loops, shared responsibility. In entrepreneurship, silence is common. Decisions are made alone. Mistakes are processed alone. Wins are often celebrated quietly, if at all.

You begin to realize that freedom comes with isolation.

There are days when no one checks in. Days when doubt creeps in because no external validation is coming. Days when you question whether the risk was worth it.

This loneliness isn't a sign you're failing. It's a sign you've stepped into ownership.

The mistake is assuming that loneliness means you should quit. In reality, it means you must develop internal confidence instead of relying on external reassurance.

Entrepreneurship Reveals Who You Really Are

More than anything else, entrepreneurship is a mirror. It reflects your discipline—or lack of it. It exposes your emotional control—or instability. It magnifies your habits. It punishes excuses brutally.

In a job, you can have off days and still get paid. In business, off days have consequences. Missed follow-ups cost money. Avoided conversations create problems. Poor decisions linger longer than you expect.

Entrepreneurship doesn't care about your intentions. It responds only to your actions. That's why many people who were "high performers" in structured environments struggle when they step out on their own. Without external pressure, they realize how much discipline was being outsourced.

The Myth of "Passive" Entrepreneurship

One of the most dangerous lies in modern business culture is the idea of passive income as a starting point.

There is nothing passive about building something from nothing.

Every successful entrepreneur you admire went through an active phase—years of learning, failing, refining, and carrying responsibility far heavier than most people realize. What looks passive later was earned through intensity earlier.

Trying to skip the active phase doesn't make you smart. It makes you unprepared.

Entrepreneurship rewards those who are willing to work when no one is watching, invest when returns are uncertain, and stay consistent when excitement fades.

Why Cash Flow Matters More than Ideas

Ideas are cheap. Execution is expensive.

Many people believe that entrepreneurship is about coming up with the right idea. In reality, it's about managing cash flow, decision-making, and endurance. A great idea with poor cash management dies quickly. A simple idea with disciplined execution survives.

Entrepreneurship forces you to understand money at a deeper level—not just revenue, but expenses, margins, timing, and sustainability. You learn quickly that growth without control creates stress, not freedom.

If you don't respect cash flow, it will control you.

The Difference Between Entrepreneurs and Hustlers

Hustling feels productive. Building feels slow. Hustlers chase activity—long hours, constant motion, endless tasks. Entrepreneurs focus on systems—processes that work even when they're not present.

Hustle is reactive.

Entrepreneurship is intentional.

At some point, you must move from doing everything yourself to building something that can operate without your constant involvement. That transition is uncomfortable because it requires trust, delegation, and patience.

Many people never make that shift. They don't own a business—they own a job they can't step away from.

Failure Is Not Optional

Failure is not a possibility in entrepreneurship. It is a certainty. The question is not whether you will fail—it's how you will respond when you do.

Some failures are loud: lost money, broken partnerships, public mistakes. Others are quiet: stagnation, missed opportunities, slow decline.

Failure teaches faster than success, but only if you're willing to examine it honestly. Ego turns failure into bitterness. Humility turns failure into education.

Entrepreneurs who survive don't avoid failure. They recover from it faster each time.

Why Entrepreneurship Requires Emotional Maturity

One of the least discussed requirements for entrepreneurship is emotional regulation.

There will be days when

- deals fall through
- clients disappear
- plans collapse
- momentum stalls.

If your emotions dictate your decisions, you will sabotage yourself. Successful entrepreneurs learn to pause. They separate feelings from facts. They avoid impulsive decisions made from fear, anger, or exhaustion.

Emotional maturity is not optional—it's foundational.

Entrepreneurship and Identity

At some point, entrepreneurship stops being something you do and becomes part of who you are. You begin to think differently. You assess risk differently. You view problems as puzzles instead of threats. You take ownership instinctively.

This identity shift is subtle but powerful.

You stop asking for permission. You stop waiting for clarity. You start moving with intention. That is when entrepreneurship becomes sustainable—not because it's easy, but because you've grown into the weight of it.

When Entrepreneurship Is Not the Answer

This needs to be said clearly:

Entrepreneurship is not the answer for everyone—and that's okay.

Some people thrive in structured environments. Some find fulfillment through leadership within organizations. Some want stability more than autonomy. Entrepreneurship is not superior. It is simply different.

Choosing not to pursue it is not a failure. Choosing it without understanding the cost is.

The Real Reward

The real reward of entrepreneurship isn't money. It's alignment. It's knowing your effort directly affects your outcome. It's building something that reflects your values. It's developing a level of self-trust most people never experience.

Entrepreneurship doesn't guarantee success—but it guarantees growth. And for those willing to carry the weight, that growth changes everything.

Closing Thought

Entrepreneurship will challenge your patience, your confidence, and your endurance. It will test your character before it ever rewards your effort. But if you approach it with honesty, discipline, and humility, it will give you something rare:

The ability to look at your life and say, *"I built this."*

CHAPTER 7

BUILDING CONFIDENCE
THAT DOESN'T BREAK

Confidence is one of the most misunderstood qualities in the world. People think confidence means being loud. They think it means never doubting yourself. They think it means walking into every room feeling sure, polished, and fearless.

That version of confidence is fragile.

Real confidence is quiet. It's steady. It doesn't need attention, validation, or approval to survive. And most importantly, it doesn't disappear the moment something goes wrong.

That's the kind of confidence you need if you want to build a life that lasts.

I didn't grow up confident. I didn't walk into rooms believing I was the smartest or the most gifted. I didn't feel secure in my position, my future, or my abilities. In fact, there were many moments where I felt like I was behind everyone else.

What I learned over time is this: confidence is not something you're given. It's something you earn.

And you don't earn it by telling yourself you're confident. You earn it by keeping promises to yourself when no one is watching.

Why Most Confidence Falls Apart

A lot of people build confidence on unstable ground. They build it on praise. When people compliment them, they feel confident. When the compliments stop, so does the confidence.

They build it on results. When things are going well, they feel confident. When they hit a setback, they question everything.

They build it on comparison. When they feel ahead of others, they feel confident. When they fall behind, they shrink.

That kind of confidence can't survive pressure.

Life will test you. Careers will challenge you. Relationships will stretch you. If your confidence depends on external validation, it will break the moment life gets uncomfortable.

Unbreakable confidence comes from internal proof.

The Difference Between Feeling Confident and Being Confident

Feeling confident is emotional. Being confident is earned. Feeling confident shows up when conditions are perfect. Being confident shows up when conditions are messy.

When I look back on the moments where my confidence truly grew, they weren't moments of success. They were moments where I showed up anyway. When I did the work even though I wasn't sure it would pay off. When I stayed disciplined even though no one was watching. When I followed through even though it would've been easier to quit.

Confidence grows when your actions tell your mind, "You can trust me."

Every time you do what you said you would do, even in small ways, your confidence strengthens. Every time you don't, it weakens.

That's why confidence isn't built overnight. It's built daily, quietly, and consistently.

Why Confidence and Discipline Are Connected

Discipline is the foundation of confidence.

People often separate the two, but they're inseparable. When you're disciplined, you don't rely on motivation. When you don't rely on motivation, you don't panic when motivation fades. When you don't panic, you stay steady.

That steadiness becomes confidence.

I learned early on that confidence wasn't something I could think my way into. I had to behave my way into it. I had to show myself, repeatedly, that I could handle discomfort, pressure, and uncertainty without falling apart.

Discipline gave me proof. Proof gave me confidence.

The Role of Failure in Confidence

Here's something most people get wrong: failure doesn't destroy confidence. Avoiding failure does.

When you avoid challenges because you're afraid of failing, you teach yourself that you're fragile. When you step into challenges and survive failure, you teach yourself that you're resilient.

Confidence grows when you realize that failure doesn't end you. Some of my most important confidence-building moments came after mistakes, setbacks, and uncomfortable lessons. Not because the failure felt good, but because I didn't run from it. I stayed in it long enough to learn.

When you know you can recover, confidence stops being fragile.

Why Comparison Kills Confidence

Comparison is one of the fastest ways to undermine confidence. The problem with comparison isn't that it shows you where you stand. The problem is that it distracts you from your own progress.

Everyone has a different timeline, a different starting point, and a different set of advantages and obstacles. When you compare your chapter one to someone else's chapter ten, you convince yourself you're behind when you're not.

Real confidence comes from competing with who you were yesterday, not who someone else is today.

When you focus on your own growth, your confidence becomes personal and stable. It's no longer dependent on where others stand.

Confidence in Corporate America and Entrepreneurship

In professional environments, confidence is often mistaken for arrogance. The truth is, confident people don't need to prove themselves constantly. They listen. They ask good questions. They stay composed.

In corporate America, confidence shows up as reliability. People trust you because you follow through. They respect you because you stay calm under pressure. They take you seriously because you don't overreact.

In entrepreneurship, confidence shows up as resilience. You don't quit at the first obstacle. You don't spiral when something doesn't work. You adjust, learn, and keep moving.

In both worlds, confidence is less about personality and more about consistency.

How to Build Confidence That Lasts

Building confidence that doesn't break requires patience and honesty.

You don't need to overhaul your life overnight. You need to start small and stay consistent. You need to identify areas where you've been breaking promises to yourself and begin repairing that trust.

Confidence grows when your words and actions align. It grows when you stop saying yes to things you won't follow through on. When you simplify your commitments. When you choose progress over perfection.

Over time, you stop questioning yourself as much. Not because you're perfect, but because you've proven you can handle imperfection.

When Confidence Becomes Identity

At some point, confidence stops being something you chase and becomes something you carry. You don't need hype. You don't need constant reassurance. You don't need to announce your plans. You trust yourself. You trust that you'll show up. You trust that you'll adjust when things don't go as planned. You trust that you can handle whatever comes next.

That's unbreakable confidence.

A Final Word on Confidence

Confidence is not about believing everything will go perfectly. It's about believing you'll handle it when it doesn't.

When you build confidence this way, it doesn't shatter under pressure. It doesn't disappear when life gets hard. It stays with you—quietly, steadily, reliably.

And that kind of confidence changes everything.

CHAPTER 8

NETWORKING WITHOUT BEING FAKE

How to Build Real Relationships
That Actually Open Doors

Networking has a bad reputation—and honestly, it deserves it. When most people hear the word "networking," they think of awkward conversations, forced smiles, business cards nobody remembers, and people pretending to care just long enough to get something. It feels transactional. Performative. Fake.

That's why so many people avoid it.

But here's the truth no one explains:

Networking is not about selling yourself.

It's about building trust.

And trust, when built the right way, changes everything.

Why Most People Get Networking Wrong

Most people approach networking with the wrong question in mind.

They ask, *"What can this person do for me?"*

That mindset shows immediately—in the way they talk, the way they listen, the way they rush the conversation toward their needs.

47

And people feel it. Even if they can't articulate why, they sense the agenda.

That's why doors stay closed.

Real networking doesn't start with asking. It starts with **curiosity**.

The people who build strong networks aren't the loudest or the most impressive. They're the ones who genuinely care about understanding others. They listen more than they talk. They ask thoughtful questions. They follow up. They remember details. They make people feel seen.

And people don't forget how you make them feel.

Relationships Move at the Speed of Trust

You cannot rush trust. You can't manufacture it. You can't fake it. You can't skip steps.

Trust is built slowly, through consistency and authenticity. It grows when people see that you show up the same way every time— not just when you need something.

This is where many young professionals struggle. They think one conversation should lead to an opportunity. One meeting should lead to a breakthrough. One introduction should change everything.

That's not how real life works.

Opportunities are usually the result of **accumulated trust**, not single interactions. People open doors for people they believe in— not people who impress them once.

The Shift That Makes Networking Natural

At some point, you have to stop thinking of networking as an event and start thinking of it as a lifestyle.

Every conversation matters.

Every interaction leaves an impression.

Every relationship has potential—not because of status, but because of humanity.

Some of the most valuable connections in your life won't look important at first. They may not have fancy titles or big platforms. But over time, relationships compound. The person you help today might be the person who recommends you tomorrow. The conversation you treat with respect today might turn into an opportunity years later.

This is why humility matters.

You never know who someone will become—or who they already are behind the scenes.

Why Authenticity Is Your Biggest Advantage

You do not need to perform to be valuable. In fact, trying too hard often works against you.

Authenticity creates comfort.

Comfort creates openness.

Openness creates trust.

When you show up as yourself—curious, respectful, grounded—people relax. Conversations flow more naturally. Walls come down. And real connection happens.

That doesn't mean oversharing or being unprofessional. It means being honest, present, and intentional.

The goal is not to be impressive.

The goal is to be **memorable for the right reasons**.

Listening Is the Most Underrated Skill in Networking

Most people are waiting for their turn to talk. Very few people are actually listening.

That's why active listening stands out immediately. When you listen fully—without interrupting, without redirecting the conversation back to yourself—you create space for trust.

People want to be heard.

People want to be understood.

When you give them that, they associate you with respect and maturity.

And respect is the foundation of every strong professional relationship.

Follow-Up Is Where Most People Fail

The conversation is only the beginning. What separates professionals from amateurs is what happens **after**.

A thoughtful follow-up message.

A reference to something specific they shared.

A genuine thank-you without an agenda.

These small actions signal seriousness and character. They show that the interaction mattered to you. Most people never follow up—which makes those who do unforgettable.

Consistency builds reputation faster than charm ever will.

Why Giving Comes Before Getting

Strong networks are built on contribution. Not grand gestures—but small, meaningful ones.

Sharing a resource.

Making a thoughtful introduction.

Offering encouragement.

Providing value without expecting immediate return.

When people see that you lead with generosity, they remember you differently. This doesn't mean overextending yourself or being used.

It means understanding that **value flows both ways over time**. The strongest relationships are reciprocal—but they don't start that way.

Someone has to go first.

Navigating Power Dynamics Without Losing Yourself

It's normal to feel intimidated when speaking to someone more experienced, more senior, or more accomplished. But confidence doesn't come from pretending you're equals—it comes from knowing your worth.

You don't need to impress powerful people. You need to respect them and respect yourself. Ask thoughtful questions. Be prepared. Speak clearly. Don't over-explain or undersell yourself.

Confidence is quiet. And people in positions of influence can sense authenticity immediately. They've seen every performance before. What stands out is sincerity.

Networks Are Built Over Years, Not Moments

This is the long game.

Relationships deepen with time, shared experiences, and mutual respect. Some connections will fade. Others will strengthen unexpectedly.

Don't measure networking success by immediate outcomes. Measure it by the quality of relationships you're building and the reputation you're creating.

Your name carries weight—whether you realize it or not.

Make sure it carries the right kind.

Final Thought for This Chapter

You don't need to become someone else to build meaningful relationships. You need to become more intentional, more present, and more genuine.

Networking done right isn't fake—it's human. And when people trust you, doors open naturally.

CHAPTER 9

MONEY MINDSET

Why Staying Broke Is Rarely About Income and Almost Always About Thinking

Money exposes what people believe. It reveals patience or impulsiveness, discipline or denial, responsibility or avoidance. Money does not create character—it magnifies it. And that's why so many people struggle with money long before they ever struggle with income.

Most young people believe the problem is not having enough money. In reality, the problem is not knowing how money works, how decisions compound, and how habits quietly shape outcomes over time. No one teaches this in school. You're taught how to earn grades, not how to earn leverage. You're taught how to memorize information, not how to manage behavior. And because of that, many people graduate financially unprepared, emotionally reactive, and vulnerable to mistakes that follow them for decades.

Money is not just math. It is mindset.

Before you ever learn how to invest, save, or grow income, you must learn how to think. Because if you're thinking stays broken, more money will not fix your life, it will accelerate the damage. I learned this early, not because I had money, but because I didn't.

Growing up, money wasn't discussed openly. It wasn't strategized. It wasn't planned. It was reacted to. Bills arrived, stress followed, and decisions were made under pressure. That environment shapes how you see money. You either learn to respect it, fear it, or avoid it entirely.

Avoidance is the most dangerous response. When you avoid learning about money, money controls you. When you delay understanding money, money punishes you later. When you outsource responsibility for your finances, you give up freedom without realizing it.

This chapter is not about becoming rich overnight. It is about not staying stuck forever. One of the biggest lies young people believe is that money problems are temporary by default. That things will "work themselves out." That someday, when income increases, discipline will magically appear. But discipline does not show up with a paycheck. It shows up with decisions. And decisions, once repeated long enough, become identity.

If you want financial freedom later, you must build financial discipline now. That does not mean deprivation. It means intentionality. It means understanding that every dollar you touch represents a choice between comfort now and freedom later. Most people choose comfort because no one ever showed them what freedom actually costs.

Debt feels harmless at first. It feels like access. Like relief. Like momentum. But debt is simply future effort being spent early, often without a plan to replace it. That is why it traps people. Not because debt is evil, but because it is easy. And easy decisions rarely lead to strong outcomes.

Spending is emotional. People spend to feel better, to fit in, to distract themselves, to cope. That's not a financial problem. That's a behavioral one. Until you understand why you spend, no budget will save you.

The most powerful shift you can make with money is learning to delay gratification without resentment. That ability alone separates people who struggle forever from people who eventually gain control.

Delayed gratification is not about denying joy. It is about choosing timing. It is understanding that short-term pleasure has long-term consequences, and long-term discipline has short-term discomfort. Everyone pays a price. You just choose when.

What school never explains is that your twenties are not about wealth—they are about habits. If you build strong habits early, money becomes a tool. If you build weak ones, money becomes a constant source of anxiety.

You do not need to earn six figures to start thinking responsibly. You need clarity, consistency, and self-respect. When you respect your future, your spending changes. When you respect your future, your choices slow down. When you respect your future, you stop making decisions that feel good for five minutes but cost you five years.

Another mistake people make is believing that saving is optional and investing is advanced. In reality, saving is stability, and investing is growth. Both matter. One protects you. The other multiplies you. Ignoring either creates imbalance.

Saving is not exciting. It does not give you status. It does not impress anyone. But it creates peace. It creates options. It creates breathing room. And breathing room allows you to think clearly instead of reacting under pressure.

Investing, on the other hand, requires patience and humility. It teaches you that progress is slow, compounding is invisible, and consistency beats intensity. The earlier you learn this, the less you rely on luck later.

Money mindset also requires understanding environment. Who you spend time with influences how you spend money. If everyone around you lives paycheck to paycheck, constant spending feels normal. If everyone around you avoids responsibility, avoidance feels justified. Your environment normalizes behavior before you ever question it.

That's why growth often requires distance. Not judgment. Distance. You cannot build a disciplined future while constantly being pulled into impulsive patterns.

Money will not save you from insecurity. It will amplify it. If you seek validation through spending, money will drain you. If you seek control through discipline, money will reward you.

The goal is not to worship money. The goal is to master it. People who master money do not obsess over it. They respect it. They understand that money represents time, energy, and choice. Once spent, time cannot be recovered. Once wasted, opportunity disappears quietly.

This is why budgeting is not restrictive—it is liberating. A budget is simply a plan that tells your money where to go instead of wondering where it went. Planning creates confidence. Guessing creates anxiety.

Another uncomfortable truth is that financial growth requires responsibility without applause. No one claps when you save. No one notices when you don't spend. No one celebrates discipline. That's why most people don't build it. They wait for recognition.

But freedom does not come from recognition. It comes from restraint. There will be seasons where you make more money. There will be seasons where you make less. But if your mindset is strong, neither season will break you. Income fluctuates. Discipline stabilizes.

You do not need to be perfect. You need to be consistent. Miss a goal, adjust. Make a mistake, correct. But never stop paying attention.

Money punishes neglect.

The earlier you accept that your financial future is your responsibility, the faster you stop blaming circumstances. Blame feels relieving in the moment, but it removes power. Ownership feels heavy, but it creates movement.

Financial literacy is not about knowing everything. It is about staying curious, staying aware, and staying honest with yourself. The goal is not control overnight. The goal is progress without regression.

Your money habits today are building the life you will live later. Whether you like that life or resent it depends on what you choose now. Money does not change who you are. It reveals whether you were prepared.

This chapter is not asking you to become obsessed with finances. It is asking you to become intentional, to stop pretending money is someone else's problem, and to stop outsourcing responsibility to "someday."

Because someday arrives faster than you think. And when it does, your habits will already be waiting.

CHAPTER 10

DISCIPLINE OVER MOTIVATION

Why Consistency Will Take You Further Than Inspiration Ever Will

Motivation is exciting. It's the spark that makes you feel unstoppable, the rush that convinces you that today is the day everything changes. Motivation shows up when a speech hits just right, when a quote resonates, when a goal feels fresh and new. It's powerful—but it's also unreliable.

Discipline, on the other hand, is quiet. It doesn't announce itself. It doesn't wait for the right mood or the perfect moment. Discipline shows up whether you feel inspired or not, whether you're confident or uncertain, whether the day feels easy or heavy. And in the long run, discipline is what separates people who talk about change from people who actually create it.

Most people build their lives around motivation. They wait to feel ready before they act. They wait to feel confident before they try. They wait to feel inspired before they commit. The problem is that life doesn't operate on feelings. Life operates on habits.

If you only act when you feel motivated, you will be inconsistent. And inconsistency is one of the fastest ways to sabotage your potential.

The Lie We're Sold About Motivation

From a young age, we're taught that success comes from passion and drive. We're told to "follow our motivation" and "wait until it feels right." What we're not told is that motivation fades quickly, especially when things get uncomfortable.

Motivation disappears when progress is slow. It disappears when results don't match effort. It disappears when life gets busy, stressful, or unpredictable. That doesn't mean you're weak. It means you're human. The mistake is assuming that successful people feel motivated all the time. They don't. They simply don't allow their feelings to dictate their actions. They move forward because they've trained themselves to act without negotiation.

Discipline is the ability to do what needs to be done even when you don't feel like doing it. It's the ability to follow through when excitement fades and reality sets in.

Discipline Is a Decision, Not a Personality Trait

Some people believe discipline is something you're born with. They look at others who seem consistent and assume they're just "wired differently." That belief is comforting because it removes responsibility—but it's also false.

Discipline is built through repetition. It's trained, not inherited.

Every time you choose to do the hard thing instead of the easy thing, discipline grows. Every time you keep a promise to yourself, discipline strengthens. And every time you break those promises, discipline weakens.

Discipline is less about intensity and more about identity. When you see yourself as someone who follows through, your behavior starts to align with that belief. Over time, discipline becomes less about forcing yourself and more about simply being who you are.

Why Discipline Feels Uncomfortable at First

Discipline feels heavy in the beginning because it requires change. It disrupts familiar patterns. It asks you to act differently than you have in the past. And change always creates resistance.

The early stages of discipline are the hardest because you don't yet trust yourself. You've likely started and stopped many times before. You've made promises you didn't keep. So, when you try again, your mind resists. It remembers past failures.

This is normal.

Discipline isn't built by making massive changes overnight. It's built by showing up consistently in small ways until trust is restored. Over time, your mind begins to believe you when you say you'll do something—and that belief becomes confidence.

Discipline Creates Freedom, Not Restriction

One of the biggest misconceptions about discipline is that it limits freedom. In reality, it creates it. Discipline gives you options. It gives you control. It allows you to move through life with intention instead of reaction.

Without discipline, you're constantly responding to circumstances. You're chasing urgency. You're putting out fires. You're living at the mercy of how you feel that day.

With discipline, you build structure. And structure creates stability. Stability creates clarity. And clarity allows you to make better decisions.

People who lack discipline often feel overwhelmed. People who have discipline feel grounded—even when life is chaotic.

The Role of Discipline in Confidence

Confidence doesn't come from positive thinking alone. It comes from evidence. Every time you follow through, you give yourself proof that you can be trusted. Every time you do what you said you would do, you strengthen your sense of self-respect. And self-respect is the foundation of real confidence.

This is why discipline is so closely tied to identity. When you act with discipline, you begin to see yourself differently. You stop questioning your ability to handle challenges because you've already proven to yourself that you can.

Confidence isn't built by avoiding discomfort. It's built by moving through it.

Why Discipline Matters More as Responsibility Grows

As life progresses, responsibilities increase. Careers demand more. Families depend on you. Time becomes limited. And when life gets busy, motivation becomes even less reliable.

Discipline is what allows you to stay consistent when life becomes complex. This is especially true in leadership, entrepreneurship, and long-term career growth. No one is coming to remind you what to do. No one is monitoring your effort. No one is checking in daily.

Discipline becomes your internal structure when external structure disappears.

The Difference Between Busy and Disciplined

Being busy is not the same as being disciplined. Busy people react. Disciplined people prioritize. Busy people fill their schedules. Disciplined people protect their time. Busy people confuse movement with progress. Disciplined people focus on what actually matters.

Discipline forces you to be honest about how you spend your energy. It pushes you to eliminate distractions and invest in what moves you forward.

Building Discipline Through Small Commitments

Discipline doesn't require dramatic transformation. It requires consistency.

Start with commitments that are small enough to keep, but meaningful enough to matter. Show up daily. Do the work even when it's boring. Build momentum through repetition.

Over time, those small commitments stack. They create rhythm. And rhythm creates reliability. Eventually, discipline becomes automatic. You stop debating whether to act—you simply act.

Discipline and Delayed Gratification

Discipline is closely tied to the ability to delay gratification. It's the willingness to sacrifice short-term comfort for long-term reward. This skill alone can dramatically change the trajectory of your life. People who can delay gratification build wealth, skills, health, and relationships more effectively. People who can't often find themselves stuck in cycles of impulse and regret.

Discipline teaches you to choose progress over pleasure, even when the tradeoff feels uncomfortable.

When Discipline Fails

There will be days you fall short. Days you break your routine. Days you don't show up the way you planned. Failure does not mean discipline is gone. It means you're human.

The key is how quickly you return.

Discipline isn't about perfection. It's about recovery. It's about refusing to let one missed day become a missed week, and one missed week become a missed year.

The Quiet Power of a Disciplined Life

Disciplined people don't need hype. They don't need external validation. They don't need constant reassurance. They trust their systems. They trust their habits. They trust themselves.

That quiet confidence is powerful. It shows up in how they speak, how they lead, and how they handle adversity.

Discipline doesn't make life easy. It makes you capable.

Final Reflection

Motivation will come and go. Discipline will stay if you train it. If you want to build a life that lasts, stop waiting to feel ready. Start acting with intention. Let discipline lead when motivation fades.

Over time, discipline will give you something motivation never can: consistency. And consistency, when applied over years, creates extraordinary results.

CHAPTER 11

PROTECTING YOUR ENERGY AND YOUR ENVIRONMENT

Why Who and What You Allow Around You Will Decide Your Future

There comes a point in life when talent, effort, and discipline are no longer the biggest determining factors in your success. At some point, **your environment takes over**.

Your environment is not just the physical space you live or work in. It is the people you spend time with, the conversations you listen to, the habits you tolerate, the standards you accept, and the energy you allow into your life on a daily basis. And whether you realize it or not, your environment is constantly shaping you.

Most people underestimate this. They think success is about doing more, trying harder, or pushing longer. And while those things matter, they eventually hit a ceiling if the environment around them is working against them.

You can have ambition, but if you are surrounded by doubt, that ambition will slowly erode. You can have discipline, but if you are constantly pulled into chaos, that discipline will be tested daily. You can have confidence, but if you are around people who subtly undermine you, that confidence will eventually crack.

This chapter is about understanding a truth that many people learn too late: **You do not rise above your environment—you are shaped by it**.

The Invisible Drain

One of the hardest things to explain to young people is why they feel exhausted even when they are not physically tired. That exhaustion often has nothing to do with work. It comes from being surrounded by the wrong energy.

Energy drains quietly. It doesn't always show up as conflict or drama. Sometimes it shows up as constant negativity, casual complaining, lack of accountability, or subtle discouragement disguised as "being realistic."

You hear it in phrases like:

"Why are you working so hard?"

"You don't need to take life that seriously."

"That's not how things usually work."

"Be careful—don't aim too high."

None of those statements sound aggressive. But over time, they chip away at your focus. They create hesitation. They introduce doubt where confidence used to live.

And if you're not careful, you begin adjusting your behavior without realizing why. You stop talking about your goals. You stop pushing as hard. You start matching the energy around you instead of maintaining your own.

This is how people slowly drift away from the life they wanted without ever making a conscious decision to quit.

Why Environment Matters More as You Grow

When you are young, your environment is mostly chosen for you. School, family, neighborhood, routine—you don't have much control. But as you get older, something shifts.

Responsibility enters the picture.

At that point, your environment becomes your responsibility. Who you keep close. Where you spend your time. What you allow to access your mind. What you tolerate emotionally. All of it becomes a reflection of your standards.

This is where many people struggle. They continue operating as if environment is accidental instead of intentional. They stay connected to people out of loyalty, habit, or comfort rather than alignment. They tolerate spaces that drain them because change feels uncomfortable. They confuse familiarity with safety.

But growth requires intentional separation.

Not from everyone.

Not dramatically.

Not angrily.

But intentionally.

The Cost of Staying in the Wrong Rooms

There are rooms that sharpen you, and there are rooms that dull you. The wrong rooms don't always look bad on the surface. They can be social. They can be familiar. They can even feel supportive at times. But pay attention to how you feel when you leave.

Do you feel energized or exhausted?

Focused or distracted?

Clear or confused?

Motivated or heavy?

Those feelings are signals.

Staying in the wrong environment has a cost, and that cost is often invisible until years have passed. It shows up as delayed progress, missed opportunities, unfulfilled potential, a quiet sense of regret.

Most people don't fail loudly. They fade quietly. And environment plays a major role in that fade.

Protecting Your Energy Is Not Selfish

There is a lie that circulates among people who struggle with boundaries: that protecting your energy is selfish.

It isn't.

Protecting your energy is responsible. You cannot build a strong future if you are constantly emotionally depleted. You cannot lead, grow, or execute at a high level if you are always recovering from unnecessary stress created by your environment.

Protecting your energy does not mean you abandon people. It means you manage access. Everyone does not deserve the same version of you. Some people get proximity. Some people get conversation. Some people get distance.

That is not arrogance. That is discernment.

As you grow, you must become more selective with what you allow into your life. Not because you think you are better than others, but because you understand where you are trying to go.

The Shift That Changes Everything

There is a moment in personal growth when you realize something powerful:

You do not need everyone to understand your journey. You just need the right environment to support it.

That realization frees you. It frees you from over-explaining. It frees you from seeking validation. It frees you from carrying other people's expectations. You stop trying to convince people of your vision and start protecting it instead.

This is maturity.

This is leadership.

This is ownership.

Creating an Environment That Supports Your Future

The environment that supports your future will often feel uncomfortable at first. It may require you to outgrow certain conversations. It may require you to change routines. It may require you to say no more often. It may require solitude at times.

But growth often feels lonely before it feels rewarding. The right environment challenges you. It stretches you. It raises your standards. It exposes your weaknesses so you can strengthen them. It encourages discipline, not comfort.

When you place yourself in environments like that, something shifts internally. Your focus sharpens. Your confidence stabilizes. Your decisions become clearer.

You stop reacting and start choosing.

Why This Chapter Matters So Much

Everything you've read up to this point in the book—belief, discipline, skill, resilience—can be strengthened or weakened by your environment. Environment amplifies who you are becoming.

If you ignore it, it will quietly work against you. If you manage it intentionally, it becomes one of your greatest advantages.

CHAPTER 12

OWNING YOUR FUTURE

From Potential to Responsibility

There comes a moment in every person's life when the excuses stop working. Not because life suddenly gets easier, but because you finally realize something deeper: no one else is responsible for where your life goes from here.

That realization can feel heavy. It can feel unfair. It can feel overwhelming. But it is also one of the most freeing truths you will ever accept.

Owning your future is not about having everything figured out. It is not about knowing the perfect career, the perfect plan, or the perfect path. It is about accepting responsibility for your decisions, your habits, and the direction you choose to move—even when clarity is incomplete.

Most people delay ownership because they believe they need certainty first. They think confidence comes before action. They think security comes before responsibility. In reality, ownership is what creates all three.

Until you own your future, you are reacting to life instead of directing it.

The Shift from Waiting to Deciding

Many young people spend years waiting.

Waiting to feel ready.

Waiting for motivation.

Waiting for approval.

Waiting for someone to tell them what to do next.

Waiting feels safe because it postpones failure. It postpones judgment. It postpones discomfort. But it also postpones growth.

When I was younger, there were plenty of reasons I could have waited. I could have waited for better grades, more confidence, more support, or clearer signs that I was "on the right path." But waiting doesn't protect you—it quietly costs you time.

Owning your future begins the moment you stop waiting for permission and start making decisions aligned with who you want to become, not who you've been so far.

This doesn't mean reckless decisions. It means intentional ones. It means choosing direction over drift.

Responsibility Is Not Blame

One of the biggest misunderstandings about ownership is that people confuse responsibility with blame.

Taking responsibility does not mean everything is your fault. It does not mean you weren't impacted by circumstances, setbacks, or unfair situations. It means you recognize that your response is still your responsibility, regardless of what happened to you.

You can acknowledge hardship without letting it define you.

Blame keeps you stuck in the past. Responsibility puts you in control of the future. When you own your future, you stop asking, "Why did this happen to me?" and start asking, "What do I do next?"

That shift alone changes how you move through life.

Practical Ownership Starts with Daily Decisions

Owning your future is not a dramatic one-time declaration. It is built through ordinary decisions made consistently over time.

It shows up in how you use your mornings.

It shows up in how you manage your money.

It shows up in how you treat your body.

It shows up in how you speak to yourself.

It shows up in who you allow to access your energy.

Most people underestimate how powerful small, repeated choices are because they don't feel important in the moment. But the future is shaped quietly. If you consistently choose comfort, your future becomes limited. If you consistently choose discipline, your future expands.

This is not theory. This is cause and effect.

Why Ownership Feels Uncomfortable at First

Ownership removes the ability to hide. When you own your future, you can no longer blame circumstances for lack of progress. You can no longer point to other people's decisions as the reason you're stuck. You must confront your habits honestly.

That discomfort is not a sign you're doing something wrong. It is a sign you are stepping into maturity.

Immature thinking says, "Someone should help me."

Ownership says, "What can I do with what I have right now?"

The second question always produces progress.

Owning Your Future in Career and Work

In your career, ownership means understanding that no company owes you fulfillment. No manager owes you growth. No role owes you purpose.

Opportunities are created by competence, consistency, and trust. When you own your future professionally, you stop asking only what the job gives you and start asking what you are building through the job. You pay attention to the skills you are developing, the problems you are learning to solve, and the reputation you are creating.

Every role teaches you something—even the ones you don't love. The difference is whether you extract the lesson or simply endure the time.

People who own their future treat every position as training for the next level, even if they don't stay there long-term.

Ownership and Entrepreneurial Thinking

You do not need to own a business to think like an entrepreneur. Entrepreneurial thinking is about being initiative. It is about seeing problems as opportunities. It is about creating value instead of waiting to be told what to do.

When you own your future, you stop seeing yourself as someone who "works for" and start seeing yourself as someone who contributes.

This mindset applies everywhere—corporate environments, nonprofits, startups, and personal life.

People who own their future do not wait for perfect conditions. They create momentum where they are.

The Role of Discipline in Owning Your Future

Discipline is the backbone of ownership. Without discipline, ownership becomes intention without follow-through.

Discipline is not about intensity. It is about reliability. It is the ability to do what needs to be done even when motivation is low. You do not need heroic effort. You need consistent effort.

When discipline becomes part of your identity, progress becomes predictable. You stop relying on bursts of inspiration and start trusting systems and routines that move you forward regardless of mood.

Owning Your Future Requires Boundaries

You cannot own your future while giving unlimited access to people, habits, and environments that drain you. Boundaries are not selfish. They are strategic.

This includes boundaries around your time, your attention, your energy, and your standards. Owning your future sometimes means saying no to things that are comfortable but unproductive. It means distancing yourself from conversations that normalize stagnation. It means choosing growth even when it feels lonely.

Every boundary you enforce protects the version of you that is still being built.

The Long View: Thinking in Years, Not Days

Most people judge progress too quickly. They expect major change in weeks when real transformation takes years.

Owning your future requires patience. It requires faith in delayed results. It requires understanding that consistency compounds quietly. You may not see the impact of your decisions immediately, but your future self will.

When you think long-term, short-term discomfort becomes easier to tolerate.

What Ownership Actually Feels Like

Ownership does not feel glamorous. It feels grounded. It feels like clarity replacing chaos. It feels like confidence replacing anxiety. It feels like direction replacing confusion.

You begin to trust yourself because you follow through. You begin to feel capable because you prove it to yourself over time.

Eventually, ownership stops feeling heavy and starts feeling empowered.

Final Reflection

Owning your future is not about perfection. It is about participation. It is about deciding that your life is worth intentional effort. It is about recognizing that you are capable of growth, even when the path is unclear.

You do not need to know every step.

You only need to take responsibility for the next one.

That is how futures are built.

CHAPTER 13

WHEN LOVE BECOMES A LIABILITY: HOW DIVORCE CAN RUIN YOU FINANCIALLY

No one gets married planning to get divorced. No one stands at the altar thinking about asset division, legal fees, custody battles, or long-term financial damage. In those moments, people think about love, commitment, partnership, and the future they believe they're building together. Divorce feels distant—something that happens to other people, other families, other lives.

But the reality is this: divorce is one of the most financially destructive events an individual can experience. And for many people, it is not the divorce itself that causes the damage, but the lack of understanding about what divorce actually costs—emotionally, mentally, and financially.

This chapter is not about discouraging marriage. It is about encouraging **awareness**. Because love without financial literacy can quietly destroy everything you've worked for.

The Hidden Financial Reality of Divorce

Divorce is often discussed emotionally. People talk about heartbreak, betrayal, stress, and pain. What is talked about far less is how divorce can reset your financial life backward by decades.

The moment a divorce begins, your financial reality changes. Two incomes often become one. One household becomes two. Shared expenses become duplicated expenses. And the lifestyle that once felt manageable suddenly becomes overwhelming.

Rent or mortgage payments increase. Utilities double. Insurance costs change. Legal fees begin accumulating immediately. Retirement accounts that once grew quietly in the background are now subject to division. Assets that took years to build can be split in months.

And none of it happens cheaply.

Divorce is expensive because conflict is expensive. Lawyers charge by the hour. Courts move slowly. Negotiations drag on. Emotions cloud judgment. Decisions made in anger or fear often cost far more than people realize until it's too late.

For many individuals, divorce doesn't just disrupt their finances—it permanently alters their financial trajectory.

When Emotion Overrides Logic

One of the most dangerous aspects of divorce is how emotion overrides logic. People who are normally rational, disciplined, and thoughtful suddenly make financial decisions fueled by anger, guilt, or the desire to "win."

People fight over assets that cost more to litigate than they are worth. They refuse reasonable compromises because of pride. They prolong legal battles because they want validation rather than resolution.

In the middle of emotional turmoil, people forget the most important rule of wealth-building: **capital preservation matters more than ego**.

Divorce exposes how unprepared many people are to separate emotion from financial decision-making. And once money is lost through legal conflict, it is rarely recovered.

The Long-Term Costs Most People Never Calculate

The financial impact of divorce does not end when the papers are signed. In many ways, that is when the real costs begin.

Child support, spousal support, and ongoing financial obligations can last years or decades. Career decisions may be limited by custody arrangements. Opportunities for relocation or advancement can disappear. Retirement timelines shift. Savings plans are delayed or abandoned entirely.

Even high earners are not immune. In fact, high earners often suffer greater losses because more assets are involved, and expectations are higher. Income that once fueled growth is now redirected toward maintaining court-ordered obligations.

The compounding effect of lost time, lost investment growth, and increased expenses can quietly dismantle financial independence.

Divorce doesn't just divide what you have. It often steals what you *could have built*.

Why Financial Misalignment Is a Leading Cause

Many divorces begin long before any legal paperwork is filed. They begin with financial misalignment. Different spending habits. Different views on debt. Different risk tolerances. Different expectations about lifestyle, savings, and future planning.

When couples do not communicate clearly about money early on, resentment builds quietly. One partner feels controlled. The other feels stressed. Financial secrecy creeps in. Trust erodes.

Money is not just numbers—it represents values, priorities, security, and control. When those values clash, conflict is inevitable.

Ignoring financial alignment does not preserve harmony. It postpones conflict until the stakes are much higher.

The Cost of Not Protecting Yourself

Many people avoid discussions about prenuptial agreements or financial boundaries because they believe it signals mistrust. In reality, it signals responsibility.

A prenuptial agreement is not a plan to fail. It is a plan to protect both parties from uncertainty. It forces honest conversations about assets, expectations, and responsibilities before emotions complicate everything.

Without protection, courts decide outcomes based on laws that may not reflect your intentions, values, or effort. Judges do not consider emotional investment. They consider statutes.

Failing to protect yourself financially does not make you more loving. It makes you more vulnerable.

Divorce and the Destruction of Momentum

One of the most overlooked costs of divorce is momentum loss. Financial success is built through consistency—steady investing, focused career growth, disciplined habits. Divorce disrupts that rhythm completely.

Time that could have been spent building skills, advancing professionally, or growing businesses is consumed by legal meetings, stress, and recovery. Mental bandwidth disappears. Focus evaporates. Productivity declines.

Even after a divorce is finalized, rebuilding takes time. Trust in relationships changes. Risk tolerance shifts. Decision-making becomes cautious or reactive.

Momentum is fragile. Divorce often shatters it.

Why This Chapter Matters to Younger Readers

If you are young and reading this, this chapter is not meant to scare you. It is meant to educate you.

Love is powerful. Commitment is meaningful. Marriage can be beautiful. But entering any long-term partnership without understanding financial consequences is reckless.

You owe it to yourself—and to any future partner—to be financially literate, emotionally mature, and strategically aware.

Marriage should enhance your life, not endanger your future.

Practical Wisdom for Protection and Prevention

The most practical step anyone can take is financial honesty—before and during a relationship. Talk about debt. Talk about goals. Talk about expectations. Talk about worst-case scenarios.

Build individual financial identity even within partnership. Understand your own credit, assets, and income. Do not outsource financial awareness to anyone else.

Seek professional advice early. Lawyers and financial planners are not just for crises. They are tools for prevention.

And most importantly, do not make life-altering financial decisions during emotional storms. Time, clarity, and perspective are invaluable assets.

The Final Truth

Divorce does not ruin people financially because they are weak. It ruins them because they were unprepared.

Prepared people make better decisions. Prepared people protect their future. Prepared people understand that love and money must coexist responsibly.

This chapter is not about fear. It is about foresight.

Because financial ruin is rarely sudden. It is usually quiet, emotional, and avoidable. And the cost of ignorance is far higher than the cost of preparation.

CHAPTER 14

WHY FINANCIAL LITERACY DETERMINES THE QUALITY OF YOUR LIFE

Money is not the most important thing in life—but it quietly touches almost everything that is. It determines where you live, how you sleep at night, the stress you carry into your relationships, the opportunities you can say yes to, and the ones you are forced to walk away from. It shapes your freedom more than people want to admit. And yet, for something that controls so much of our day-to-day reality, financial literacy is rarely taught with intention, honesty, or urgency.

Most people are introduced to money through confusion. They grow up watching adults argue about it, stress over it, or avoid talking about it altogether. Bills arrive in the mail like silent threats. Debt becomes normalized before it is understood. Credit cards are framed as freedom, not obligation. And by the time real financial responsibility shows up, most people are already behind.

Financial illiteracy doesn't announce itself loudly. It doesn't crash through the door. It creeps in quietly. It looks like living paycheck to paycheck even as income rises. It looks like constantly feeling behind despite working hard. It looks like being afraid to open bank statements. It looks like staying in jobs, relationships, or situations you've outgrown because the math doesn't allow you to leave.

That is why financial literacy is not just about money. It is about control. When you understand money, you gain leverage over your life. When you don't, money becomes a source of fear, pressure, and reactionary decision-making. And the truth is, no amount of motivation, ambition, or talent can compensate for a lack of financial understanding over time.

One of the greatest lies young people are told is that money will "figure itself out later." That somehow, once you earn more, everything will fall into place. But earning more without understanding money often just means making bigger mistakes with more zeros attached to them. Income does not fix ignorance. It magnifies it.

Financial literacy begins with awareness. It begins the moment you stop treating money as something that happens to you and start treating it as something you manage intentionally. That shift alone separates people who feel trapped from people who feel empowered.

Most people never stop to examine the emotional relationship they have with money. They don't ask why they spend the way they do, why saving feels uncomfortable, or why certain purchases provide temporary relief but long-term stress. Money habits are rarely logical. They are learned, absorbed, and repeated. They are often rooted in childhood experiences, family patterns, and unspoken beliefs about worth, security, and success.

Without literacy, money becomes emotional. It becomes something you react to rather than plan for. You spend when you feel stressed. You avoid numbers when they make you uncomfortable. You delay decisions because facing reality feels overwhelming. Over time, avoidance turns into damage.

Understanding money gives you clarity. It replaces fear with facts. It allows you to see where you are, not where you wish you were. And while that honesty can be uncomfortable at first, it is the foundation of every meaningful financial turnaround.

Financial literacy teaches you how to think long-term in a world obsessed with immediacy. It helps you understand that most financial pain does not come from one bad decision but from hundreds of small, unexamined ones made consistently over time. It shows you that discipline is more powerful than income, and that freedom is built gradually, not suddenly.

One of the most practical benefits of financial literacy is choice. When you understand your numbers, you are no longer guessing. You know what you can afford. You know what you cannot. You know the cost of saying yes and the consequences of saying no. That clarity removes panic from decision-making.

People without financial literacy often feel rushed. They make emotional decisions under pressure because they don't know where they stand. People with financial literacy move slower and with more confidence. They are not immune to stress, but they are less reactive. They don't need to guess.

Another overlooked aspect of financial literacy is how deeply it affects relationships. Money problems are one of the leading causes of conflict in marriages, partnerships, and families. Often, it's not the lack of money that causes the damage, but the lack of communication and understanding around it. When one person understands the financial reality and the other avoids it, resentment grows. When both avoid it, chaos follows.

Financial literacy creates a shared language. It allows couples and families to plan together instead of blaming each other. It turns money from a weapon into a tool. And it prevents small issues from becoming irreversible fractures.

The absence of financial literacy also keeps people stuck in cycles they don't understand. They wonder why they can't get ahead, why progress feels temporary, or why financial emergencies always seem to hit at the worst time. Without understanding cash flow, savings buffers, and risk management, every unexpected expense feels catastrophic.

Literacy does not eliminate problems, but it reduces their impact. It prepares you for reality instead of leaving you exposed to it.

One of the most empowering aspects of financial literacy is that it removes mystery. Money stops feeling like a force you can't control and starts feeling like a system you can learn. You don't need to be a math expert. You don't need to be wealthy. You need to be willing to learn, track, and adjust.

Understanding basic concepts like budgeting, debt, interest, investing, and risk changes the way you see the world. You start recognizing traps instead of falling into them. You stop being impressed by appearances and start paying attention to fundamentals. You realize that many people who look successful are financially fragile, while others who live quietly are building real security.

Financial literacy also protects your future self. It allows you to make decisions today that reduce pressure tomorrow. It creates margin. Margin is the difference between panic and patience. It is the space that allows you to absorb setbacks without collapsing.

Without margin, every disruption feels like a crisis. With margin, challenges become manageable. Perhaps the most important reason financial literacy matters is that it aligns your money with your values. When you don't understand your finances, money controls your priorities. When you do, you get to decide what matters most. You can choose where to invest your time, energy, and resources intentionally.

That might mean prioritizing stability over status. It might mean choosing flexibility over luxury. It might mean building slowly instead of chasing fast wins. Whatever the choice, literacy gives you the power to choose consciously instead of drifting.

Financial literacy does not promise wealth. It promises awareness. And awareness is what allows growth to happen.

No one is born financially literate. It is not a reflection of intelligence or character. It is a skill. And like any skill, it improves with attention, practice, and humility. The most dangerous mindset is believing it's too late or unnecessary. The most powerful mindset is deciding to learn now.

If you take nothing else from this chapter, understand this: money will touch every major decision you make in your adult life. Avoiding it does not protect you. Understanding it does.

Financial literacy is not about greed. It is about responsibility—responsibility for yourself, responsibility to the people who depend on you, responsibility for the future you haven't met yet.

When you learn how money works, you stop fearing it. When you stop fearing it, you stop making desperate decisions. And when you stop making desperate decisions, your life begins to stabilize in ways that compound over time.

That is why financial literacy is not optional. It is foundational. It does not guarantee success, but without it, success becomes fragile. And with it, even modest resources can be turned into long-term security, flexibility, and peace of mind.

Money will never replace purpose. But when handled well, it supports it. And that is what makes financial literacy one of the most important skills you will ever develop.

CHAPTER 15

BETTING ON YOURSELF

There comes a moment in every person's life when the noise fades just enough for the truth to surface. It doesn't arrive dramatically. There's no soundtrack, no spotlight, no applause. It shows up quietly, usually after disappointment, frustration, or exhaustion. It arrives when you realize that waiting for permission has gotten you nowhere, that hoping someone else will rescue you has left you standing still, and that playing it safe has cost you more than taking risks ever did.

That moment is when you understand that the most important bet you will ever place is not on a job, a company, a relationship, or an opportunity. It is on yourself.

Betting on yourself is not reckless optimism. It is not arrogance. It is not pretending you have all the answers. Betting on yourself is a decision made in uncertainty. It is choosing to trust your ability to learn, adapt, and endure when outcomes are unclear. It is the refusal to outsource your future to someone else's approval.

Most people never make that bet. They wait for conditions to be perfect. They wait to feel ready. They wait until confidence magically appears. They wait until the risk feels smaller. And while they wait, time moves forward without them. Opportunities close. Skills stagnate. Regret quietly accumulates.

What no one tells you is that readiness is a myth. Confidence is built *after* commitment, not before it. The people you admire most didn't feel ready when they stepped forward. They felt afraid, uncertain, and exposed. What separated them from everyone else was not certainty—it was willingness.

I learned this slowly, not through one dramatic leap, but through a series of moments where comfort and growth demanded opposite choices. There were times when staying put felt easier. Times when the paycheck felt safer than the dream. Times when explaining why I didn't try would have been simpler than explaining why I failed. And in each of those moments, I had to confront the same question: Do I trust myself enough to figure it out?

Betting on yourself does not mean you believe you are special. It means you believe you are capable of becoming better. It means you understand that skill can be developed, mistakes can be corrected, and setbacks are not verdicts. It means you are willing to take responsibility not just for success, but for failure as well.

That responsibility is what scares people.

When you bet on yourself, you remove excuses. You no longer get to blame the system, the timing, the economy, or the lack of support. You own the outcome. If it works, it's on you. If it doesn't, it's also on you. That level of accountability is uncomfortable, and most people would rather complain from the sidelines than step into the arena.

But here's the truth: avoiding responsibility does not protect you. It only delays the inevitable realization that no one else was ever going to live your life for you.

There is a quiet cost to not betting on yourself. It shows up years later in conversations that start with, "I almost…" or "I could have…" or "I wish I had…" It shows up in resentment toward people who took chances. It shows up in bitterness disguised as realism. It shows up in a life that looks fine on the outside but feels unfinished on the inside.

When you bet on yourself, you accept uncertainty in exchange for possibility. You accept discomfort in exchange for growth. You accept temporary instability in exchange for long-term fulfillment. That tradeoff is not glamorous, and it is rarely linear. There will be moments when you question your decision, when progress feels slow, when doubt resurfaces. That does not mean you made the wrong choice. It means you are in the middle of becoming.

One of the biggest misconceptions about betting on yourself is that it requires burning bridges or making reckless moves. It doesn't. Often, it starts quietly. It starts with choosing discipline over distraction. It starts with investing time into learning instead of numbing. It starts with saving instead of spending, practicing instead of procrastinating, speaking up instead of shrinking back. The bet compounds through consistent actions long before it shows visible results.

People often ask when they'll know it's working. The answer is uncomfortable: you won't at first. The early signs are internal, not external. You'll notice that you trust your judgment more. You'll notice that setbacks don't derail you as easily. You'll notice that you stop seeking validation for every decision. Those changes matter more than immediate wins because they signal that your identity is shifting from dependent to self-directed.

Betting on yourself also forces you to confront fear honestly. Not fear as an abstract idea, but fear as a daily presence. Fear of failing publicly. Fear of disappointing others. Fear of being wrong. Fear of starting over. These fears do not disappear when you commit to yourself. They walk with you. The difference is that they no longer drive.

Courage is not the absence of fear. It is the willingness to act while fear is present. Every meaningful step forward carries risk, and every risk carries the possibility of loss. The people who build lives they are proud of are not immune to this reality. They simply decide that the cost of inaction is higher than the cost of trying.

As this book comes to a close, I want you to understand something deeply: betting on yourself is not a one-time decision. It is a practice. You will be asked to make this choice again and again—when things go well and when they don't, when support is strong and when it disappears, when momentum is high and when it stalls. Each time, the question will be the same: Will you trust yourself enough to keep going?

CHAPTER 16

YOU ARE WHAT YOU EAT

Why Your Diet Is Quietly Shaping Your Energy, Your Mind, and Your Future

No one tells you this when you're young, but the way you eat is one of the most powerful decisions you make every single day. Not because food is trendy. Not because nutrition is fashionable. But because food quietly determines how you think, how you feel, how you perform, and how long you can sustain the life you say you want.

When people talk about success, they talk about mindset, discipline, work ethic, and ambition. Rarely do they talk about what fuels all of it. Yet the truth is unavoidable: your body is the vehicle that carries every dream you have. If that vehicle is neglected, under fueled, or abused, everything else suffers.

School never taught you this. No one explained that your energy levels, focus, emotional stability, immune system, and long-term health are directly connected to what you eat. Instead, food was framed as convenience, reward, comfort, or entertainment. Eat what tastes good. Eat what's fast. Eat what's cheap. Eat now, deal with the consequences later.

Later always comes.

Most people don't realize how much food controls their life until they feel constantly tired, unfocused, irritable, or sick. They blame stress. They blame work. They blame age. They blame everything except the daily choices that are quietly stacking up in their body. Food doesn't punish you immediately. It waits. And by the time people feel the damage, habits are already deeply rooted.

Eating isn't just physical. It's behavioral. It's emotional. It's cultural. It's learned. And because no one ever teaches you how to eat intentionally, most people eat on autopilot. They eat what they grew up eating. They eat what their friends eat. They eat what marketing tells them to eat. And then they wonder why their body feels like it's working against them.

Your body is never working against you. It's responding to what you give it.

The human body is remarkably intelligent. It adapts. It compensates. It survives. But survival is not the same as thriving. When you feed your body poorly, it doesn't shut down overnight. It does what it can with what it's given. Over time, though, the cracks show. Energy drops. Focus fades. Motivation becomes harder to access. Recovery slows. Stress feels heavier. Sleep gets worse. Inflammation rises. Mood swings increase.

People assume these things are normal. They are common, but they are not normal. What you eat becomes the raw material for everything your body builds: cells, hormones, neurotransmitters, muscle, immune defenses, even the chemistry of your brain. When the inputs are low-quality, the outputs will be, too. No amount of motivation can override biology forever.

This matters even more if you are building something—a career, a business, a family, a legacy. High performance demands high-quality fuel. You would never pour cheap fuel into a high-performance engine and expect it to run optimally. Yet people do exactly that with their bodies every day and expect focus, discipline, and endurance in return.

Food is not just fuel for your body. It is fuel for your decisions.

When your blood sugar spikes and crashes, your patience drops. When your gut is inflamed, your mood suffers. When your body is undernourished, your brain struggles to concentrate. When your diet lacks nutrients, your stress tolerance shrinks. These aren't character flaws. They're physiological responses.

This is where the phrase "you are what you eat" stops being a cliché and starts being a reality. You don't just become what you eat physically. You become it mentally and emotionally as well. A diet built on processed foods, sugar, and constant stimulation creates a body that is inflamed and reactive. A diet built on whole foods, balance, and intention creates a body that is stable, resilient, and capable.

Most people chase productivity hacks while ignoring the foundation. They want better focus without better nutrition. They want more energy without better habits. They want clarity while feeding their body confusion. The irony is that the simplest changes often create the biggest shifts.

Eating well is not about perfection. It's about awareness. It's about recognizing that every meal is either helping you or hurting you. There is no neutral. Even when you think food doesn't matter, your body is keeping score.

One of the biggest lies people believe is that eating healthy is complicated. It's not. It has been made complicated. Marketing, trends, and extremes have distorted something that should be intuitive. Your body responds best to real food. Food that looks like it came from the earth, not a factory. Food with ingredients you can pronounce. Food that nourishes rather than overstimulates.

Another lie is that eating healthy means deprivation. In reality, poor eating is what deprives you. It deprives you of energy, clarity, longevity, consistent performance, and confidence in your own body. People confuse discipline with restriction, but discipline is freedom. When you eat intentionally, you free yourself from energy crashes, constant cravings, and the emotional rollercoaster that comes with poor nutrition.

The relationship you have with food often mirrors the relationship you have with yourself. People who respect their body fuel it differently than people who abuse it. People who value long-term outcomes make different choices than people chasing short-term comfort. Food exposes priorities.

This doesn't mean you never enjoy a meal. It means enjoyment is intentional, not constant. It means food is a tool, not a coping mechanism. It means you stop using food to numb stress, boredom, or emotion and start using it to support the life you are building.

Eating well is also about self-respect. When you choose foods that support your health, you are sending yourself a message: my body matters. My future matters. My ability to show up matters. That message compounds over time. It builds identity. You start to see yourself as someone who takes care of their body, and that identity spills into other areas of life.

Your diet also affects how long you can stay in the game. Success is rarely about intensity alone. It's about sustainability. Burnout doesn't only come from working too hard. It comes from asking too much of a body that isn't supported. People push themselves relentlessly, ignoring nutrition, sleep, and recovery, then act surprised when their body forces them to slow down.

Your body will always collect its debt. You can pay it daily with good habits, or you can pay it later with illness, fatigue, and limitation.

One of the most overlooked aspects of nutrition is its impact on mental health. Anxiety, depression, and brain fog are not always purely psychological. The gut and brain are deeply connected.

Inflammation, nutrient deficiencies, and blood sugar instability can all influence mood and cognition. When people clean up their diet, they are often shocked by how much calmer and clearer they feel. Not because life changed, but because their internal environment did. Eating well doesn't solve every problem, but it makes problems easier to face.

This chapter isn't about telling you what to eat. It's about teaching you to think differently about food. To see it as leverage. To see it as strategy. To see it as an investment rather than an afterthought.

You don't need extreme diets. You don't need obsession. You need consistency and awareness. You need to ask better questions. How does this food make me feel afterward? Does it give me energy or take it? Does it help me focus or make me sluggish? Does it support my goals or sabotage them?

When you start paying attention, your body gives you clear answers. Food is one of the few things you engage with multiple times every day. That makes it powerful. Small decisions, repeated consistently, shape outcomes more than big decisions made occasionally. Eating is a daily vote for the kind of life you want.

People who eat intentionally often find that other habits improve as well. Sleep gets better. Exercise becomes easier. Discipline strengthens. Confidence grows. Momentum builds. That's not accidental. It's alignment.

Your body wants to work with you. It wants to heal, adapt, and perform. But it needs the right inputs. You cannot starve your body of nutrients and expect abundance in your life.

This is what they didn't teach you in school: success is physical as much as it is mental. You cannot separate the two. Your body is not a side project. It is the foundation.

When you eat with intention, you are betting on your future self. You are choosing clarity over chaos, energy over exhaustion, longevity over short-term pleasure. You are choosing to be someone who can carry their ambition without breaking.

And that is the kind of choice that compounds for a lifetime.

CHAPTER 17

WINNING THE WAR IN YOUR MIND

There is a battle happening inside you every single day. It doesn't make noise. It doesn't leave bruises. No one else can see it. But it is the most important battle you will ever fight because every outcome in your life is decided there first. Long before money is made or lost, long before relationships succeed or fall apart, long before confidence shows up in the way you walk into a room, the result has already been determined in your mind.

Most people spend their lives trying to fix the outside of their lives without ever addressing the inside. They chase better circumstances, better opportunities, better connections, better timing. They believe that once something external changes, everything internal will fall into place. But the truth is the opposite. Your inner world shapes your outer world. Your thoughts shape your habits. Your habits shape your decisions. Your decisions shape your life.

Winning the war in your mind is not about positive thinking or pretending everything is okay. It is about learning how to control your internal dialogue instead of letting it control you. It is about understanding how fear, doubt, insecurity, comparison, and past experiences quietly influence your behavior, often without you realizing it. And it is about developing the discipline to interrupt destructive thought patterns before they turn into destructive outcomes.

The reason this war matters so much is because the mind is powerful, but it is also lazy. Left unchecked, it defaults to comfort, safety, and familiarity. It will convince you to stay where you are, even when where you are is costing you your future. It will rationalize bad decisions. It will replay old failures. It will exaggerate fear and minimize potential. And if you allow it, it will talk you out of the very life you claim you want.

This is why intelligence alone is not enough. Plenty of smart people stay stuck. Plenty of talented people never reach their potential. Plenty of capable people live small lives. The difference between those who rise and those who remain stagnant is not ability. It is mental control. It is the ability to manage thoughts instead of being managed by them.

At some point in life, you realize that your biggest enemy is not the system, your upbringing, your lack of resources, or other people. Your biggest enemy is the voice in your head that tells you to quit, to settle, to wait, or to play it safe. That voice is subtle. It often sounds reasonable. It disguises itself as logic, realism, or self-protection. But more often than not, it is fear wearing a familiar mask.

Fear shows up in many forms. Sometimes it looks like procrastination. Sometimes it looks like perfectionism. Sometimes it looks like overthinking. Sometimes it looks like self-sabotage just when things are about to improve. Fear rarely announces itself openly. Instead, it whispers doubts, magnifies risks, and minimizes your ability to handle adversity. If you never learn to recognize it, fear will quietly dictate the direction of your life.

One of the hardest truths to accept is that your mind will lie to you. It will tell you that you are not ready, even when you are more prepared than you think. It will tell you that others are ahead, even when comparison serves no purpose. It will tell you that failure would be devastating, even though failure is often the greatest teacher you will ever have. Winning the war in your mind begins when you stop assuming that every thought you have is true.

Thoughts are not facts. Feelings are not instructions. Just because something feels uncomfortable does not mean it is wrong. Just because something feels scary does not mean it should be avoided. Growth often feels threatening because it requires change, and the brain is wired to resist change. Understanding this alone can free you from years of unnecessary self-doubt.

Your mind is constantly looking for evidence to support whatever belief you already hold. If you believe you are behind, your mind will find examples to confirm it. If you believe you are incapable, your mind will highlight every mistake. If you believe you are capable of growth, your mind will start noticing opportunities. This is why belief is not just motivational language. It is a mental filter that determines what you see and how you interpret your experiences.

Many people carry mental baggage they never unpack. Old failures. Harsh words spoken years ago. Moments of embarrassment or rejection. Experiences that planted seeds of insecurity. Over time, these moments form narratives, and those narratives become identities. You stop saying, "I failed" and start saying, "I am a failure." You stop saying, "That didn't work" and start saying, "I'm not good at this." Without realizing it, you allow past moments to define present decisions.

Winning the war in your mind requires revisiting those narratives and questioning them. Not denying them but reframing them. Failure does not mean you are incapable. It means you learned something. Rejection does not mean you are unworthy. It means someone else made a decision based on their own perspective. Embarrassment does not mean you should shrink. It means you survived discomfort and lived to grow from it.

One of the most dangerous mental traps is waiting to feel confident before taking action. Confidence is not a prerequisite for action. Confidence is the result of action repeated over time. If you wait until fear disappears, you will wait forever. Courage is not the absence of fear; it is the decision to move forward despite it. Every time you act in alignment with your values instead of your emotions, you strengthen your mental resilience.

Another silent enemy in the mind is comparison. In a world fueled by social media, it is easier than ever to measure your progress against carefully curated versions of other people's lives. Comparison distorts reality. It convinces you that you are behind without showing you the full picture. It ignores context, timing, and individual paths. The moment you measure your worth against someone else's highlight reel, you surrender control of your mental state.

The truth is, you are not supposed to have the same life, timeline, or journey as anyone else. Your job is not to outrun others. Your job is to become who you are capable of becoming. Winning the war in your mind means learning to focus inward instead of outward. It means tracking your own progress, setting your own standards, and competing with who you were yesterday, not with someone you barely know.

Mental strength is built through repetition, not inspiration. Just like physical strength, it develops through consistent effort over time. Each time you choose discipline over comfort, you reinforce a new pattern. Each time you redirect a negative thought, you weaken its grip. Each time you do what you said you would do, even when it is inconvenient, you build trust with yourself. That trust is the foundation of mental toughness.

You cannot control every thought that enters your mind, but you can control which ones you entertain. The mind is like a room with many doors. Thoughts will knock constantly. You decide which ones get invited in and which ones are turned away. This takes awareness and practice. At first, you will notice negative thoughts after they have already affected you. Over time, you will begin to catch them earlier. Eventually, you will stop many of them before they take root.

Silence is an underrated weapon in this war. Constant noise leaves no space for reflection. When you never slow down, you never hear what is driving your behavior. Creating moments of stillness allows you to observe your thoughts instead of being swept away by them. This is where clarity lives. This is where patterns become visible. This is where growth begins.

Winning the war in your mind also means learning how to talk to yourself. Your internal dialogue matters more than external feedback. If you speak to yourself with contempt, you will move through life with hesitation. If you speak to yourself with honesty and encouragement, you will build momentum. This does not mean ignoring weaknesses. It means addressing them without self-destruction. Constructive self-talk leads to improvement. Destructive self-talk leads to paralysis.

There will be days when your mind is heavy. Days when motivation feels distant. Days when doubt feels louder than belief. Winning does not mean those days disappear. Winning means you no longer let those days dictate your identity or your future. You show up anyway. You do the work anyway. You keep moving forward, even when progress feels invisible.

Over time, this consistency changes you. You become someone who trusts yourself. Someone who does not panic under pressure. Someone who can sit with discomfort without running from it. Someone who understands that thoughts are temporary, but decisions have lasting consequences.

The war in your mind never fully ends. New challenges bring new doubts. New levels bring new fears. But each battle you win strengthens you for the next one. Each time you choose discipline over distraction, truth over comfort, growth over ease, you prove to yourself that you are capable of more than your mind initially allows.

This chapter is not about becoming fearless. It is about becoming aware. It is about recognizing that your mind can either be your greatest ally or your greatest obstacle. And the difference lies in how intentionally you train it.

When you learn to master your thoughts, you stop being reactive and start being deliberate. You stop drifting and start directing. You stop surviving and start building. And once you win the war in your mind, the battles outside become far more manageable. Because the strongest position you can ever stand in is this: knowing that no matter what happens around you, you are in control of how you respond.

And that control changes everything.

CHAPTER 18

MAN UP AND TAKE CARE OF YOUR KIDS

Even When Life Doesn't Work Out the Way You Planned

There are few responsibilities heavier, more sacred, and more defining than being a parent. No career achievement, no financial milestone, no public success will ever outweigh the role you play in the life of your children. Yet this is one of the most uncomfortable truths society avoids saying plainly: Many people are willing to fight harder for their pride, their freedom, or their comfort than they are willing to fight for their kids. This chapter exists to confront that reality honestly, without sugarcoating it, and without apology.

Life does not always work out the way you planned. Relationships fail. Marriages end. Circumstances change. People grow apart. What does not change, however, is the responsibility you carry once you bring a child into this world. Parenthood is not conditional on your happiness, your relationship status, or how fairly you believe life has treated you. When things fall apart between adults, children do not suddenly need you less. In fact, they need you more.

One of the most damaging lies people tell themselves is that showing up financially is enough. Money matters, yes. Providing stability matters. But presence matters just as much, if not more.

Children are not spreadsheets. They do not measure love solely through checks or court-ordered obligations. They measure it through consistency, effort, emotional safety, and the quiet reassurance that someone is not going anywhere no matter how messy life becomes.

Being a parent means choosing responsibility even when it is inconvenient. It means choosing maturity over ego. It means understanding that your children did not ask to be born into broken circumstances, adult conflict, or unresolved resentment. They did not choose the tension, the distance, or the silence. They only experience the outcome. And over time, those experiences shape how they see themselves, how they trust others, and how they show up in the world.

When relationships end, it becomes tempting to retreat inward. People justify absence with excuses that sound reasonable on the surface. They say the situation is complicated, that communication is difficult, that emotions are high, that the timing is not right. But children do not experience complexity the way adults do. They experience presence or absence. They experience effort or neglect. They experience consistency or unpredictability. Over time, those patterns become their emotional blueprint.

Showing up for your kids does not mean being perfect. It does not mean having all the answers. It means being willing to do the uncomfortable work of staying engaged even when the relationship with the other parent is strained. It means refusing to weaponize your children as leverage in adult conflicts. It means choosing to protect them from emotional crossfire instead of pulling them into it.

There is a quiet strength in reliability. A child who knows you will call when you say you will call, show up when you promise to show up, and listen when they speak grows up with a deeper sense of security. That security becomes confidence. Confidence becomes resilience. And resilience becomes the foundation for a healthier adult life. You may never see the immediate impact of your consistency, but the absence of it will always leave a mark.

Too often, people confuse masculinity or independence with detachment. They believe being strong means being unaffected, distant, or emotionally guarded. In reality, strength shows up in responsibility. Strength shows up in patience. Strength shows up in doing what needs to be done even when no one is applauding you for it. Taking care of your kids is not weakness. It is one of the most demanding forms of leadership there is.

This responsibility extends beyond logistics. Children watch how you handle adversity. They watch how you speak about the other parent. They watch how you respond to frustration, disappointment, and stress. Even when you think they are not paying attention, they are absorbing everything. The way you carry yourself during difficult seasons teaches them how to handle their own challenges later in life.

When you disappear emotionally or physically, children internalize it. They rarely assume it has something to do with adult circumstances. More often, they assume it has something to do with them. Over time, that internalized absence can turn into self-doubt, abandonment wounds, or a belief that love is conditional. These are not abstract consequences. They show up later in relationships, self-worth, and emotional regulation.

Taking care of your kids also means taking care of yourself. You cannot show up well if you are constantly running from responsibility or numbing yourself to avoid discomfort. Growth as a parent often requires confronting your own patterns, your own unresolved pain, and your own emotional habits. This is difficult work. But avoiding it only ensures that the same cycles repeat.

There is also a financial reality that cannot be ignored. Raising children requires stability, planning, and long-term thinking. Irresponsible financial behavior does not just hurt you. It affects your children's sense of safety and opportunity. Teaching them discipline, accountability, and respect for money starts with how you manage your own obligations. Being present but unstable is not enough. Providing financially but being absent is not enough either. Both matter.

At some point, maturity requires letting go of the narrative that life owes you ease. Parenthood is not about fairness. It is about duty. It is about recognizing that your children did not choose you, but you chose the actions that brought them here. That choice carries lifelong responsibility, regardless of how circumstances evolve.

Man up does not mean suppressing emotion. It means handling it responsibly. It means choosing restraint over reaction, commitment over convenience, and presence over escape. It means showing your children that accountability does not disappear when life becomes uncomfortable.

Years from now, your children will not remember every detail of what you said or did. They will remember how you made them feel. They will remember whether you showed up when it mattered. They will remember whether you were someone they could rely on, even when things were not easy.

This chapter is not about guilt. It is about clarity. You cannot control every outcome in life, but you can control your effort. You can control your integrity. You can control whether you choose responsibility or avoidance. Taking care of your kids is not something you do when it is convenient. It is something you do because it is right.

If you want to leave a legacy that actually matters, start there.

CHAPTER 19

MANIFESTING YOUR LIFE

How Your Thoughts Quietly Shape the Future You End Up Living

Manifestation is one of the most misunderstood concepts of our time. For some, it has been reduced to slogans, vision boards, and wishful thinking. For others, it feels abstract or unrealistic, something reserved for people who believe in luck or fate rather than effort and discipline. The truth is far less dramatic and far more powerful. Manifestation is not magic. It is not about sitting still and hoping the universe delivers what you want. Manifestation is about alignment. It is about how your thoughts, beliefs, and internal narratives quietly shape the decisions you make, the actions you take, and ultimately the life you live.

Whether you realize it or not, you are already manifesting your life every single day. The question is not whether manifestation works. The question is whether you are doing it intentionally or unconsciously. Most people manifest by default. They allow their fears, insecurities, past failures, and external influences to dictate their expectations, and those expectations guide their behavior. Over time, behavior becomes habit, habits become identity, and identity becomes destiny. That is manifestation in its most basic and undeniable form.

From a young age, you are taught to focus on what is directly in front of you. You are trained to react rather than to envision. School teaches you how to follow instructions, meet requirements, and wait for approval. What it does not teach you is how powerful your internal world is in shaping your external reality. No one explains that the way you speak to yourself, the stories you repeat in your mind, and the beliefs you accept as truth quietly influence every major outcome in your life. By the time most people realize this, they are already living a life they did not consciously choose.

Your thoughts are not harmless background noise. They are instructions. They tell your brain what to look for, what to avoid, and what to believe is possible. When you repeatedly think that you are behind, not good enough, or incapable, your brain works tirelessly to prove you right. It filters opportunities, conversations, and experiences through that belief system. You hesitate where you should act. You stay quiet where you should speak. You settle where you should push. Over time, the life you live becomes evidence of the thoughts you once entertained.

Manifestation begins with awareness. You cannot change what you do not notice. Most people go through life allowing their thoughts to run unchecked, shaped by their upbringing, their environment, and their past experiences. They mistake these thoughts for facts. They assume that because a thought feels familiar, it must be true. In reality, many of the beliefs you carry were never chosen by you. They were absorbed. They were repeated. They were normalized. And because they were never questioned, they became invisible.

When you begin to pay attention to your internal dialogue, you may be surprised by how often it works against you. You may notice how quickly your mind jumps to worst-case scenarios, how easily it dismisses your goals as unrealistic, and how often it reminds you of what went wrong instead of what is possible. This is not a personal failure. It is conditioning. The mind is designed to protect you, not to propel you forward. It prioritizes comfort and certainty over growth and possibility. Manifestation requires you to override that instinct.

This does not mean ignoring reality or pretending challenges do not exist. It means choosing which narrative you allow to dominate your thinking. There is a difference between acknowledging obstacles and allowing them to define you. When you consciously decide to focus on growth, solutions, and long-term vision, you begin to send a different set of instructions to your mind. You start asking better questions. Instead of asking why something will not work, you ask how it could. Instead of assuming rejection, you prepare for opportunity. These shifts may feel subtle, but over time they compound into massive change.

Your beliefs act as a ceiling. They determine how high you are willing to reach and how much discomfort you are willing to tolerate in pursuit of your goals. If you believe success is reserved for others, you will unconsciously sabotage your own progress. If you believe you are capable of learning, adapting, and improving, you will persist longer, recover faster, and take more calculated risks. Manifestation is not about instant results. It is about sustained alignment between what you believe and how you act.

One of the most powerful aspects of manifestation is identity. You do not rise to the level of your goals; you fall to the level of your identity. If you see yourself as someone who quits when things get hard, you will eventually quit, no matter how strong your initial motivation is. If you see yourself as someone who follows through, adapts, and figures things out, you will behave accordingly, even when motivation fades. Identity-driven behavior is consistent because it feels natural. Manifestation becomes effortless when your actions align with who you believe you are.

This is why visualization, when done correctly, is so effective. Visualization is not about fantasizing. It is about rehearsing. When you consistently imagine yourself showing up as disciplined, confident, and prepared, your brain begins to treat that version of you as familiar. Familiarity reduces resistance. Actions that once felt uncomfortable start to feel normal. Over time, you stop forcing yourself to act differently because the behavior matches your self-image. That is manifestation taking root.

Your environment plays a critical role in this process. The people you spend time with, the content you consume, and the conversations you engage in all influence your thought patterns. If you surround yourself with negativity, complacency, or constant doubt, it becomes significantly harder to maintain a forward-focused mindset. This does not mean cutting everyone out of your life. It means being intentional about what you allow to shape your thinking. Manifestation thrives in environments that support growth, accountability, and belief.

Manifestation also requires patience. We live in a culture that celebrates immediate results and overnight success stories, while quietly ignoring the years of alignment and effort that preceded them. When results do not show up quickly, people assume manifestation does not work and abandon the process. In reality, the delay is often where the transformation happens. While you are waiting for external results, your internal foundation is being built. Your mindset is shifting. Your habits are forming. Your resilience is strengthening. When the opportunity finally arrives, you are ready to meet it.

It is important to understand that manifestation does not eliminate struggle. In many cases, it invites it. When you decide to think differently, act intentionally, and pursue a higher standard for your life, you will encounter resistance. Old habits will push back. People may question your choices. Doubt will resurface. This is not a sign that you are doing something wrong. It is a sign that you are breaking away from patterns that once kept you small. Growth always comes with friction.

One of the most overlooked elements of manifestation is responsibility. Manifestation is empowering because it places control back in your hands, but that control comes with accountability. If your thoughts shape your actions, and your actions shape your outcomes, then you must take ownership of where you are and where you are going. This does not mean blaming yourself for everything that has happened. It means recognizing that you have more influence over your future than you were ever taught to believe.

As you begin to consciously shape your thoughts, you will notice changes in how you approach challenges. Problems become puzzles rather than roadblocks. Setbacks become feedback rather than proof of failure. You start to see patterns where you once saw chaos. This shift does not make life easier, but it makes it clearer. Clarity is powerful because it allows you to move with intention instead of reacting emotionally.

Manifestation is not separate from discipline. In fact, discipline is one of its most practical expressions. When you believe in a future version of yourself, discipline becomes an act of respect. You show up not because you feel like it, but because you are committed to becoming someone who does. Over time, discipline reinforces belief, and belief reinforces discipline. This cycle is what turns vision into reality.

The life you are living today is the result of thousands of small decisions made over time. Those decisions were influenced by what you believed was possible, appropriate, or necessary. By changing your internal narrative, you begin to change the quality of those decisions. You choose differently. You respond differently. You invest your time and energy more intentionally. Slowly, almost imperceptibly, your external world begins to reflect your internal shift.

Manifestation is not about controlling every outcome. It is about controlling your input. You cannot dictate every circumstance you face, but you can decide how you interpret and respond to them. That response determines whether a challenge becomes a dead end or a turning point. When you trust yourself to adapt and grow, uncertainty becomes less intimidating. You stop waiting for perfect conditions and start building momentum with what you have.

As this book comes to a close, understand this: the power to shape your life has always been within you. It was never missing. It was simply unused. You were taught to look outward for answers when the most influential work was always internal. By choosing your thoughts carefully, aligning your actions with your values, and committing to growth even when it is uncomfortable, you begin to manifest a life that reflects your potential rather than your fears.

Manifestation is not about becoming someone else. It is about becoming more fully yourself. It is about removing the limitations you once accepted and stepping into the responsibility of creating a life that feels intentional, grounded, and meaningful. When your thoughts, actions, and values align, progress becomes inevitable.

The future you want is not waiting for you somewhere down the road. It is being shaped by what you choose to believe today, by how you act when no one is watching, and by whether you are willing to bet on yourself even when certainty is absent. When you understand this, manifestation stops being a concept and becomes a way of living.

And once you begin living this way, you will realize something powerful: the life you once imagined is no longer something you are hoping for. It is something you are actively building, one thought, one decision, and one disciplined action at a time.

CHAPTER 20

FINAL WORD

There comes a moment in every life when the noise quiets just enough for the truth to speak.

Not the loud truth that comes from social media, expectations, or pressure. Not the truth shaped by fear or comparison but the quieter truth that lives underneath everything else—the one you feel when you're alone with your thoughts, when no one is watching, when you're honest with yourself.

That truth usually sounds something like this:

I'm meant for more than the life I'm currently living.

Not more in the sense of fame or money or attention—but more meaning, more ownership, more alignment. More control over your time, your decisions, and your future. More integrity between who you are and who you're becoming.

If you've read this far, that truth has already been whispering to you for a long time.

And now it's time to stop ignoring it.

For most of your life, you were taught to wait. Wait your turn. Wait to be chosen. Wait until someone tells you that you're ready. Wait until you feel confident. Wait until you have enough experience, enough money, enough clarity, enough certainty.

Waiting feels responsible. Waiting feels safe. Waiting feels like maturity. But waiting is also how people quietly give up on themselves. Not all at once. Not dramatically. Slowly. Respectably. One delayed decision at a time.

They don't quit on their dreams—they postpone them. They don't abandon their potential—they shrink it until it feels manageable. They don't betray themselves in obvious ways—they do it subtly, by choosing comfort over courage again and again.

And one day, they wake up and realize that the life they're living is not the life they would have chosen—but it's the life they settled into.

This book was written to interrupt that path. Because the truth is, you don't need permission anymore. You don't need validation from people who don't live the life you want. You don't need approval from systems that were never designed to maximize your potential. You don't need to wait until the fear disappears or the confidence magically shows up.

Confidence is not the requirement. Commitment is.

You are not ready because you feel fearless. You are ready because you are willing to grow. And growth has never required certainty—it has only ever required honesty and action.

Most people believe their future exists somewhere ahead of them, as if it's a destination they'll eventually arrive at if they just keep moving. But that's not how life actually works.

Your future is not waiting for you. It is being constructed, quietly and relentlessly, by the decisions you make today. Every conversation you avoid. Every habit you keep. Every excuse you tolerate. Every time you choose what's easy over what's right. Every time you delay the hard thing you know you need to do.

Those moments don't feel significant in isolation. But compounded over time, they become your life.

The same is true in the opposite direction. Every uncomfortable decision. Every moment of discipline. Every boundary you set.

Every risk you take despite fear. Every time you show up when it would be easier not to.

Those moments build something, too.

They build self-trust.

And self-trust changes everything.

When you trust yourself, you stop outsourcing your confidence. You stop waiting for permission. You stop looking outside for answers that only you can live into. You move differently. You decide faster. You recover quicker. You take responsibility without resentment.

Betting on yourself doesn't mean you believe you're perfect or guaranteed to win. It means you're willing to take ownership even when the outcome is uncertain. It means you stop protecting yourself from failure and start protecting your potential from neglect. It means you accept that you might fail—and choose to move anyway.

That choice is terrifying for some people. For others, it's liberating. For most, it's both. Because betting on yourself forces you to confront the one thing you can't escape: accountability.

No one else to blame. No one else to rescue you. No one else to take responsibility for the life you're building.

That's heavy. But it's also powerful.

When you own your choices, you also own your progress. When you own your mistakes, you also own your growth. When you own your direction, you reclaim your agency. And agency is what most people are truly searching for, even if they don't know how to name it.

They don't want an easier life. They want a life that makes sense. A life where effort connects to outcome. A life where they can look in the mirror and respect the person staring back.

That respect doesn't come from perfection. It comes from alignment. From knowing that you're not hiding from your potential. From knowing that you're not playing small to keep others comfortable. From knowing that even when things are hard, you're choosing forward movement over stagnation.

The world will try to convince you that betting on yourself is reckless. That it's naive. That it's selfish. That it's irresponsible. But the truth is, living a life you don't believe in is far more dangerous. It drains your energy. It dulls your ambition. It turns your gifts into regrets. And it teaches the people watching you—especially your children—that safety is more important than purpose.

You don't need to have everything figured out to move forward. You just need to stop pretending that staying still is the responsible option. Growth has always required risk. Integrity has always required courage. And meaningful lives have always been built by people who were willing to choose themselves even when it felt uncomfortable.

Not in an arrogant way. In an honest way. In a way that says, *I will take responsibility for my life, even if it scares me.*

That's what this book has been leading you toward. Not motivation. Not hype. Not empty inspiration. Ownership.

You are not behind. You are not late. You are not broken.

You are early—if you choose to act now.

And if there's one thing I want you to carry with you after you close this book, it's this:

No one is coming to give you permission.

No one is coming to hand you confidence.

No one is coming to live your life for you.

But you are here.

You are capable.

And you are allowed to bet on yourself.

So do it. Quietly if you must. Imperfectly if you have to. Slowly if that's all you can manage. Just don't ignore the truth any longer. Your future is not something you wait for. It is something you build.

And it starts now.

ABOUT THE AUTHOR

Thomas Hightower was born in Hartford, Connecticut and raised in Stafford Springs, Connecticut, where early doubts and limitations shaped his relentless drive to prove that circumstances do not define destiny.

He graduated from Norfolk State University with a Bachelor of Arts in Interdisciplinary Studies, earning a full scholarship in track and field and cross country. During his collegiate career, Thomas became an 8-time All-Conference athlete, exemplifying discipline, resilience, and leadership both on and off the field.

By the age of thirty, Thomas rose to an executive role within a multi-billion-dollar company, defying expectations once placed on him as a student and athlete. Today, he is the proud owner of six businesses, while also working full-time at Zoom Communications, where he continues to lead, build, and innovate.

Above all, Thomas is a devoted father to his daughters, Gianna and Ava, who inspire his commitment to legacy, growth, and purpose.

Through his writing, mentorship, and leadership, Thomas is dedicated to helping the next generation develop confidence, discipline, and ownership—the tools required to succeed in the real world long after school ends.

Email the author at tomhigh23@gmail.com for feedback.